ERIC MOSKOW, M.D.,
AND TOM BIRACREE

HEART SMART

A Doctor's Commonsense Guide to
Understanding Cholesterol and
Saving Your Heart

•

ST. MARTIN'S PRESS   NEW YORK

*To Ricki, Elliot, Hillary, Melanie, and Jeremy—
the hearts of my life.*

—E. S. M., M.D.

As always, for Nancy and Ryan.
—T. L. B.

HEART SMART: A DOCTOR'S COMMONSENSE GUIDE TO UNDERSTANDING CHOLESTEROL AND SAVING YOUR HEART. Copyright © 1995 by Eric Moskow and Tom Biracree. All rights reserved. Printed in the United States of America. No part of this book may be used or reproduced in any manner whatsoever without written permission except in the case of brief quotations embodied in critical articles or reviews. For information, address St. Martin's Press, 175 Fifth Avenue, New York, N.Y. 10010.

Design by Pei Loi Koay

Library of Congress Cataloging-in-Publication Data

Moskow, Eric.
   Heart smart : a doctor's commonsense guide to understanding cholesterol and saving your heart / Eric Moskow and Tom Biracree.
      p. cm.
   "A Thomas Dunne book."
   ISBN 0-312-13085-6
   1. Coronary heart disease—Popular works. 2. Cholesterol—Popular works. I. Biracree, Tom, 1947– . II. Title.
RC685.C6M68   1995
616.1'2305—dc20   95-15986
                                                                                              CIP

First Edition: October 1995

10 9 8 7 6 5 4 3 2 1

ACKNOWLEDGMENTS

This project sprouted from the creative mind of Tom Dunne; we're grateful to him and to Tony Seidl, who brought us all together. Thanks to everyone at Family Medical Associates, especially David, Wendy, and Marjorie. We much appreciate the patience and editorial guidance provided by Neal Bascomb. Finally, we would like to pay tribute to the American Heart Association for its tireless efforts to educate the public and physicians about heart disease while rallying massive research that may eventually conquer America's leading killer.

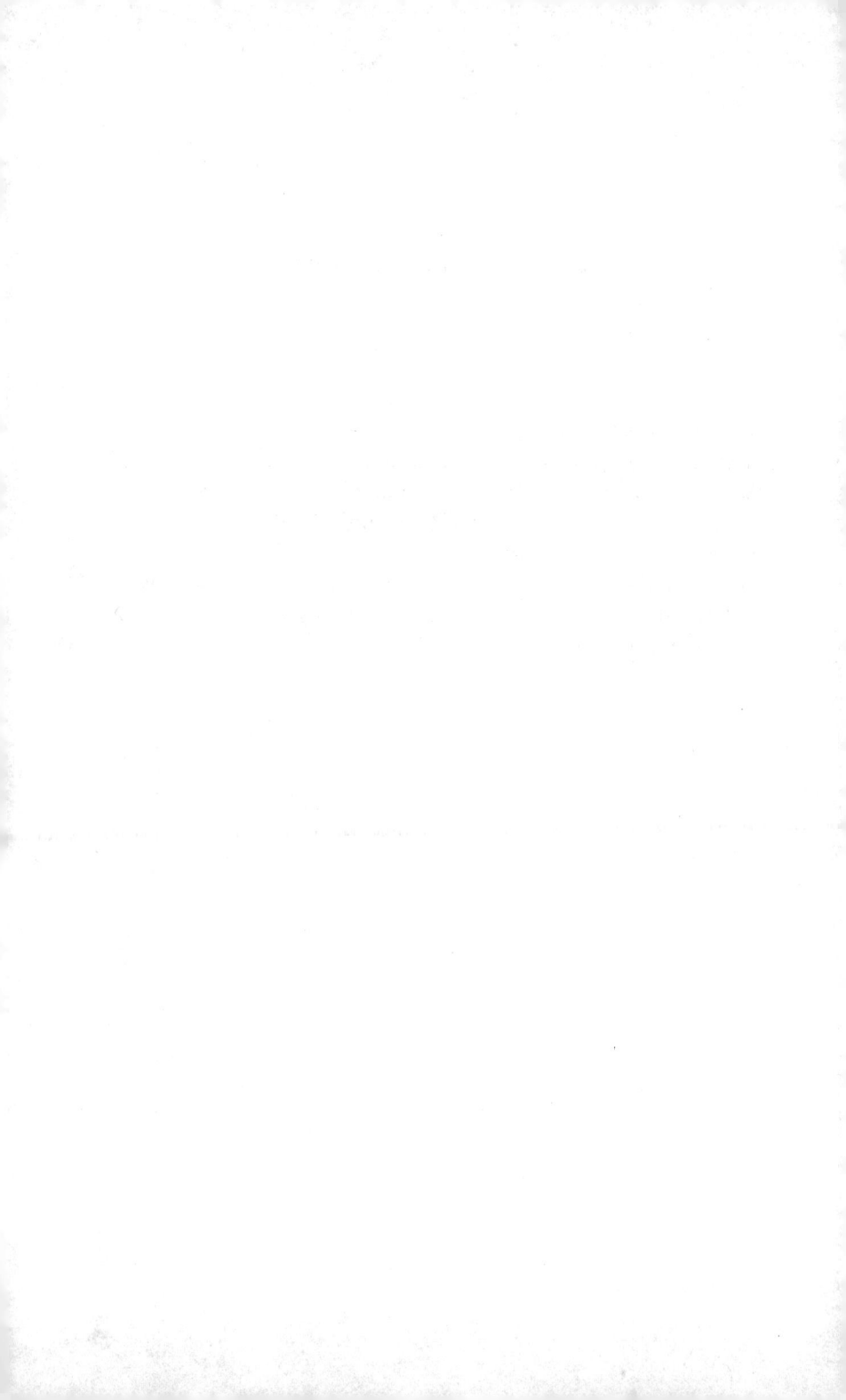

CONTENTS

Acknowledgments	v
Introduction: Cholesterol and Common Sense	1

PART 1: Everything You Need to Know About Cholesterol and Your Personal Cholesterol Risk — 5

1: The ABC's of Cholesterol	7
2: Testing Your Cholesterol—Do It Now!	13
3: What You Should Know About Your Total Cholesterol Level	19
4: Looking at Your Lipoproteins	23
5: Summing Up Your Cholesterol Risks	28

PART 2: Cholesterol—What Hurts and What Helps — 31

6: Why Do So Many of Us Have a Cholesterol Problem?	33
7: The Cholesterol Villains and Heroes	38
8: Villain #1—Dietary Cholesterol	42
9: Villain #2—Saturated Fat	45
10: Villain #3—Smoking	48
11: Villain #4—Stress	51
12: Villain #5—Obesity	53
13: Hero #1—Polyunsaturated Fats	57
14: Hero #2—Monounsaturated Fats	59
15: Hero #3—Fish	61
16: Hero #4—Exercise	63

17: Hero #5—Soluble Fiber	**66**
18: Hero #6—Alcohol	**70**

PART 3: It's Your Choice—A Flexible, Sensible, Ten-Step Cholesterol-Reduction Plan — **73**

19: Commit to a Lifetime of Heart-Smart Choices	**75**
20: Your Exercise Options	**80**
21: Decision Making at the Supermarket	**87**
22: Cholesterol-Melting Breakfasts	**100**
23: Healthful Lunches	**106**
24: Nutritious and Delicious Dinners	**112**
25: Sensible Snacking	**119**
26: Savvy Menu Selections When Dining Out	**122**
27: Opt for a Stress-Reducing Lifestyle	**128**
28: Decide on a Long-Term Heart Health Monitoring Program	**133**

PART 4: When Lifestyle Changes Aren't Enough — **135**

29: Cholesterol-Lowering Drugs	**137**
Appendix 1: Cholesterol and Children	**142**
Appendix 2: Fat and Cholesterol Content of Selected Foods	**144**

INTRODUCTION

Cholesterol and Common Sense

This book begins with one fact and one promise:

FACT: The vast majority of Americans can add healthy, productive years to their lives by lowering their blood cholesterol levels.

PROMISE: If you give me a couple hours of your time, I'll explain everything you need to know about cholesterol, help you assess your risk of developing coronary artery disease, and show you simple choices you can make to significantly reduce that risk.

I decided to write this book because I long ago gave in to the occupational hazard of being a family doctor—most of my patients became my friends. I knew their spouses, their children, what they did for a living, and a lot of other personal history that was often very valuable in diagnosing and treating their medical problems.

The downside was the personal as well as professional anguish I felt when I had to rush to their homes or the hospital in the middle of the night for a life-threatening emergency—most often a heart attack or stroke that ripped a friend of mine away from his loved ones when he or she should have been enjoying the best years of life.

> **A SOBERING FACT**
>
> In one-third of all cases, the first sign of coronary artery disease is sudden death.

What made these deaths more tragic was the fact that the coronary artery disease that causes most premature heart attacks and a significant percentage of strokes can be prevented. In 1994, the American Heart Association convention heard the results of a landmark study on the effects of lowering blood cholesterol. The results, which Nobel Prize–winning cardiologist Dr. Michael Brown called "absolutely astonishing," proved beyond a doubt that reducing blood cholesterol levels not only reduces the risk of heart attacks but also saves lives.

However, at that same convention, an American Heart Association panel reported that more than 75 percent of all physicians neglect their patients' welfare by failing to tell them how lowering cholesterol levels can lengthen their lives. The study showed that only 22 percent of patients were aware of their risk factors and only 24 percent had ever done *anything* to reduce their blood cholesterol levels.

Most of my patients knew their cholesterol levels. But I wasn't doing an effective job of making them aware of what their risk factors were and exactly how those risks could be substantially reduced—or even eliminated.

My solution was to invite my patients into my office for a lengthy chat after hours, when the phone wasn't ringing off the hook. At first, I had to twist a few arms—everyone expected a lecture. But I was far more interested in answering questions than in preaching.

I began with one statistic: **Every 1 percent reduction in total blood cholesterol means at least a 2 percent reduction in the risk of having a heart attack.** After learning a little bit about cholesterol, all my patients could begin to make a few different choices in their lifestyles that would begin to lower their heart attack risk *the very next day*. By applying some common sense to their diets and lifestyles over a few months, most of my patients achieved 20 to 50 percent risk reductions. Over time, I found myself called to fewer heart attack victims in the middle of the night.

Word of my after-hour chats spread quickly, but a growing patient load cut down on the time I had for them. Eventually, I realized that the only way I could educate enough people was to turn my discussion into a book.

This book is called *Heart Smart: A Doctor's Commonsense Guide to Cholesterol and Saving Your Heart* because it contains everything everyone really needs to know about cholesterol, written in language everyone can understand. This book concentrates on facts, not fads. Most important, it contains a wealth of practical tips everyone can implement to make his or her life longer and healthier.

This book is not a diet or exercise program! Millions of dollars have been spent on research studies that proved something almost all of us already knew—in the long run, diets don't work. The reason is that diets tell instead of teach. We may last a day, a week, even a month, but eventually we all grow weary of having someone else tell us what to eat. We all want to make our own—and better—choices.

How do we accomplish that goal? By becoming educated consumers of food. We already know that making the best choice in cars, houses, electronics, jewelry, clothing, and other products requires schooling ourselves in the basics and lots of comparison shopping. The same is true with our diet and lifestyle—the more we know, the easier it is to make the most intelligent day-to-day decisions.

In just a couple of hours, you'll be an educated consumer when it comes to cholesterol. And your life will be better and probably longer for the effort.

1

EVERYTHING YOU NEED TO KNOW ABOUT CHOLESTEROL AND YOUR PERSONAL CHOLESTEROL RISK

1

THE ABC'S OF CHOLESTEROL

WHAT IS CHOLESTEROL?

Cholesterol is a white, waxy fatty substance. In its purest form, a pile of it would look and feel a lot like a pile of Ivory Snow flakes. If you had enough cholesterol, you could use it to put a nice shine on your car. Lanolin, which is used as a lubricant, a leather protectant, and a cosmetics ingredient, is really cholesterol taken from sheep's wool.

These white, waxy flakes were extracted from gallstones by a Frenchman named Poulletier de la Salle in 1784. Gallstones are hard pellets that form in the gallbladder, a small pouch that stores bile produced by the liver and squirts it into the small intestine to help digestion. It's not surprising that scientists soon discovered that cholesterol traveled in bile—in fact its name means "bile solid" in Greek.

Gallstones can cause extreme pain when they clog the gallbladder duct, the first hint that cholesterol can be a troublemaker. But it wasn't until the twentieth century that we began to understand where cholesterol came from and its complex roles in our body chemistry.

BLOOD CHOLESTEROL LEVELS AND RISK OF DEATH

The Multiple Risk Factor Intervention Trial, which followed 356,222 men ages thirty-five to fifty-seven for six years, found that higher blood cholesterol levels increase the risk of death from heart attack.

Blood Cholesterol	Deaths per 1,000 Men
140	3
180	4
200	5
240	8
260	10
280	13
300	18

SURPRISE—OUR BODIES MANUFACTURE CHOLESTEROL

We hear so many bad things about cholesterol that it's logical to assume that it's manufactured in clandestine laboratories and delivered to the back doors of fast food restaurants in unmarked fifty-five-gallon drums.

The truth is that cholesterol isn't toxic waste but a substance that's essential to life. Not only do our livers manufacture it, but so do the livers of all other animals. That's why cholesterol is present in eggs, milk, meat, and fish. Because plants don't have livers, there's no cholesterol in vegetables, fruits, or grains.

"Jeopardy" Answer: Our Livers and the Foods We Eat

"Jeopardy" question: Where does the cholesterol in our bloodstream come from? For a person with an average diet, three-quarters of the cholesterol used by the body is made by the liver; the rest comes from animal products we eat.

> **SOME DEFINITIONS YOU SHOULD KNOW**
>
> **Atherosclerosis** A condition in which plaque deposits build up on the walls of arteries.
>
> **Coronary Artery Disease** Atherosclerosis in the arteries that supply blood to the heart. It is considered serious when the artery is narrowed 50 to 70 percent.
>
> **Heart Attack** A complete or almost complete blockage of a coronary artery that results in damage to the heart muscle. Coronary artery disease is the cause of almost all heart attacks.
>
> **Angina pectoris** An intense pain and tightening in the chest that reduces the amount of oxygen available to the heart because of coronary artery disease. Angina is often triggered by exertion or stress.
>
> **Stroke** A complete or almost complete blockage of an artery that supplies blood to the brain.

CHOLESTEROL'S VERY IMPORTANT JOBS

Our bodies use cholesterol in two basic ways. First, like other waxes, it protects. Cholesterol is used to make the membrane or "skin" that envelops every cell in our body. It helps insulate our entire nervous system so our brains can communicate with the rest of our bodies ("Foot, stamp on that ant now!"). And it's secreted through our pores to soften and protect our skin.

Second, cholesterol is an ingredient used by the body in the production of bile acids, which travel along with cholesterol in bile, a yellow fluid produced by the liver, which is essential to the digestion of fatty foods in the intestines; several hormones, including estrogen, testosterone, and progesterone; and vitamin D, which is important for strong bones.

CHOLESTEROL HAS TO BE PACKAGED FOR THE JOURNEY TO OUR CELLS

Our bodies can't directly use the cholesterol that we manufacture and eat. It's a kind of fat called a "lipid," which doesn't dissolve in the main constituent of blood—water. When you try to wash fats, oils, or grease from your hands with just water, it doesn't work. You need soap, which breaks down the fats and allows them to be washed away. Since we don't have soap in our system, the job of converting cholesterol into substances that can travel to the cells falls upon the liver.

The human liver—the largest organ in our body—acts like a food packaging and distribution center. Its solution to the cholesterol problem it to wrap the lipids in proteins (called "lipoproteins"), which allows them to be carried through the bloodstream.

NOT ALL CHOLESTEROL IS THE SAME

The remarkably talented liver puts cholesterol into two different packages. Most of it is combined with fats called "triglycerides" into little units called "very-low-density lipoproteins," or VLDLs. The remainder becomes "high-density lipoproteins," or HDLs.

VLDLs Become LDLs

As the VLDLs travel through the body, the triglycerides are absorbed by the cells to burn as energy or to store as fat. What's leftover are "low-density lipoproteins," or LDLs, made up largely of cholesterol. LDLs contain the cholesterol that our bodies need.

In 1958, the Nobel Prize for Medicine was awarded to two University of Texas scientists who discovered that many cells of our bodies have special receptors that attract and capture LDLs so the cholesterol can be extracted. About 20 percent of these docks for cholesterol are in cells throughout the body that use it to manufacture protective membranes or hormones; the other 80 percent are in the liver, which extracts cholesterol to make bile acids and to eliminate excess cholesterol from the bloodstream.

OUR GROSS NATIONAL PRODUCT

What are we Americans best at producing? According to the 1990 National Health and Nutrition Examination Survey, it's extra girth around our waistlines. Despite growing evidence that the risk of heart attack can be slashed by lowering blood cholesterol levels and body weight, the percentage of Americans classified as obese grew an amazing 8 percent between 1980 and 1990. A smaller study conducted at the same time showed a 6 percent increase in average cholesterol levels.

The National Institutes of Health define as obese any man who weighs 24 percent more than the weight range considered ideal and any woman who is 20 percent above that level. By these criteria, the percentage of overweight Americans includes:

33 percent of white females
32 percent of white males
50 percent of Mexican-American and African-American females

The health prospects for the future look equally bleak. According to a 1994 National Institutes of Health study, the percentage of adults who exercise regularly plummeted from 42 percent in 1991 to 32 percent in 1994. Because exercise is vital in maintaining high HDL cholesterol levels and lowering LDL levels, the lazy majority's risk of heart disease will rise.

Too Many LDLs Means T.R.O.U.B.L.E.

LDLs are like teenagers. If there are enough activities to keep them busy, they're happy and productive. But if there's not enough for them to do, they start to hang out in groups on street corners and get into trouble.

Excess LDLs are likely to cause a problem if they're allowed to hang out in the bloodstream. The same chemical properties that make it easy for LDLs to dock with receptors also enable it to stick to the walls of blood vessels. When the LDLs circulating in the bloodstream greatly exceed the receptors, the LDLs tend to adhere to certain blood vessels, hardening into a substance called plaque. If an imbalance between LDLs produced and LDLs used or eliminated continues for many years, plaque can seriously restrict blood flow in an artery, causing chest pains called "angina." A plaque buildup can completely cut off blood flow, causing a heart attack or a stroke.

HDLs Are the Good Guys

In tracking patients over the course of decades, researchers have conclusively established that the higher the level of HDLs, the less trouble the excess LDLs cause. What scientists haven't determined is exactly how HDLs do their good deeds. HDLs may somehow make it more difficult for LDLs to adhere to artery walls; HDLs may also act like janitors, helping to sweep stray LDLs from the bloodstream and into the liver for disposal. At the very least, the more cholesterol packaged in HDLs, the less ends up in LDLs.

CAN YOU HAVE TOO LITTLE CHOLESTEROL?

Too little total cholesterol is seldom a problem except in cases of severe malnutrition. But nearly two-thirds of all adult Americans have one or more of the following problems:

- Too much total cholesterol
- Too many LDLs
- Too few HDLs

That's why it's vital that you find out your blood cholesterol levels and assess your risk of developing coronary artery disease.

2

TESTING YOUR CHOLESTEROL—
DO IT NOW!

Suppose I called you into my office and said, "I've got some bad news and some good news. The bad news is that you're scheduled to die today. The good news is that if the price is right, I might be able to get you a few more years." I suspect that you'd be willing to put up everything you owned to continue living.

Now, back to real life. I have only good news—I can help you get those extra years and the down payment is less than a hundred bucks. That money is for the first essential step in controlling cholesterol—getting a good cholesterol test to determine your current level of risk.

CHOLESTEROL TESTING—IGNORANCE IS NOT BLISS

If I recommended not looking at your bank balances for years, you'd say I was nuts. Yet eight out of ten American adults have no idea what kind of deposits are building up on the walls of their arteries. Studies show only about half of all adults have ever had a cholesterol test and less than 20 percent remember the results.

THE NATIONAL CHOLESTEROL EDUCATION PROGRAM TESTING GUIDELINES

The National Cholesterol Education Program established by the National Institutes of Health recommends that every adult over age twenty have his or her total cholesterol level tested. A total cholesterol level test is quick and easy (it requires just a single drop of blood from a prick of your finger) and doesn't require fasting. The NCEP recommends that everyone who hasn't had his or her total cholesterol tested for a significant length of time go to a physician or medical laboratory for testing that includes determining HDL level. The NCEP also recommends that adults who have been diagnosed with coronary artery disease also have a lipoprotein analysis, a more comprehensive test.

There's a new, inexpensive, accurate home cholesterol testing kit on the market that makes determining your total cholesterol level one of the easiest and most convenient of all medical procedures. Unfortunately, the home cholesterol test doesn't give you your HDL cholesterol level or a lipoprotein analysis.

THE HEART-SMART RECOMMENDATION

Every adult should know three important numbers:

- Total cholesterol level
- HDL level
- Ratio of total cholesterol to HDLs

Every adult—not just those who have already developed heart disease—also should have a lipoprotein analysis that produces two additional results:

- Triglyceride level
- LDL level

The more comprehensive cholesterol testing isn't significantly more expensive, painful, or difficult to prepare for. A small vial of blood will be drawn from a vein instead of a drop from your finger. Also, accurate triglyceride measurement requires fasting for twelve to fourteen hours—the most convenient schedule is to have dinner

HOME CHOLESTEROL TESTING

Johnson & Johnson's Advanced Care Cholesterol Test has made determining your total cholesterol easy and inexpensive. The test kit, which retails for under $20, consists of:

- A test cassette
- A results chart
- A lancet to prick your finger
- A gauze pad and a bandage
- An instruction booklet
- A question and answer booklet

The company also maintains a toll-free help line staffed by nurses to answer questions.

The testing procedure is simple. You prick a finger, then place one or two drops of blood in a small well on the test cassette. After waiting two minutes, you pull a tab to start the test. In ten to twelve minutes, the end of the test window turns green, indicating that the test is complete. You read the results like a thermometer, then consult a chart to translate the reading to a total blood cholesterol level.

Although home testing is a great way to check your progress, you should not rely on one result to determine your risk of heart disease. You and your physician should determine your risk level after a complete lipid profile done by a professional laboratory.

NOTE: The home test is not for use by hemophiliacs, people under age twenty, or those on blood-thinning medication.

---

around 6 or 7 P.M. the night before, then schedule a test first thing the next morning before eating breakfast. (No coffee before the test—sorry.) The more information you have, the more accurately you can assess your health risks and decide on the appropriate lifestyle changes to reduce those risks.

Caution: You shouldn't be tested when you are or have recently been seriously ill, if you're pregnant, or if you've had a baby in the last three months. A number of medications can also affect your cholesterol levels, including oral contraceptives, beta-blockers, steroids, and estrogen. If you're in doubt about whether a test is appropriate, ask your doctor.

HOW ACCURATE ARE CHOLESTEROL TESTS?

Federal guidelines call for a margin of error of no more than 3 percent, which means that a total cholesterol level of 200 really means a range from 194 to 206. The home cholesterol test manufactured by Johnson & Johnson meets this standard. But not all medical and hospital laboratories follow the strict procedures necessary to achieve this level of accuracy. Because of machine and human error, tests done at clinics, health fairs, and even doctors' offices can vary widely in quality.

So what should you do? I suggest two prudent steps:

- Have your cholesterol testing done by a physician you trust. I spend a lot of time training my staff and selecting laboratories to ensure the best possible testing.
- Accept your test results as a very good estimate, not a number carved in stone. As I discuss shortly, what's important about testing is placing you in a range of low risk, moderate risk, or high risk.

WHAT SHOULD YOU DO WITH YOUR TEST RESULTS?

Sit down with your doctor to discuss the results of your cholesterol testing in light of your overall health. Your risk of having a heart attack or stroke can obviously be affected by any other existing heart problems, a family history of heart disease, diabetes, smoking, and a host of other conditions.

However, many physicians don't have the time or the inclination to discuss cholesterol test results in great detail. That's why I discuss in some detail the current information we have about what the results of cholesterol testing mean for adults who are otherwise in good health.

HOW IS CHOLESTEROL MEASURED?

When physicians refer to cholesterol levels, we're talking about the cholesterol that's circulating through your arteries and veins, so the test requires drawing some blood. Since cholesterol is a solid, we measure its weight—in milligrams, a tiny unit of measure (if you break open an antibiotic capsule, the contents probably weigh 500 milligrams). Blood, a liquid, is measured in deciliters, a tenth of a liter or about 3 ounces.

Blood cholesterol is always measured in milligrams per deciliter (abbreviated as mg/dl) For example, your total cholesterol might be 200 mg/dl. To make this book easier to read, I'll drop the mg/dl from now on.

WHERE DOES THE INFORMATION ON THE HEALTH RISKS OF CHOLESTEROL COME FROM?

The risk levels I discuss in this book come from the best kind of scientific studies—taking a very large group of people, accurately

---

MEET YOUR CIRCULATORY SYSTEM

No machine works as long and as hard as your heart and the rest of your circulatory system.

- Your heart beats more than thirty million times per year, or more than a billion times by your fortieth birthday.
- All the arteries, veins, capillaries, and other vessels of your circulatory system measure about sixty thousand miles in length.
- In your lifetime, your heart will pump more than one million barrels of blood.
- Your blood brings energy and oxygen to three hundred trillion cells with every heartbeat.

testing their cholesterol levels on a regular basis, then computing how many people at each level die of heart disease over a long period of time. The most famous, and one of the best, was the Framingham Heart Study, which has followed nearly 4,000 residents of Framingham, Massachusetts, since 1948. Another, the Multiple Risk Factor Intervention Trial, focused on 360,000 men in eighteen U.S. cities for six or more years. These massive efforts, and many others, have produced results so similar that we can be quite sure they are accurate.

3

WHAT YOU SHOULD KNOW ABOUT YOUR TOTAL CHOLESTEROL LEVEL

•

Total cholesterol is the most easily measured and by far the most talked about test result. It is also probably the most misunderstood. Simply meeting the widely publicized federal goal for total blood cholesterol doesn't mean that you've eliminated your risk of developing coronary artery disease. On the other hand, many people with high test readings don't realize how dramatically they can lower their heart attack risk with even modest total blood cholesterol reductions.

TARGET = 200

For most of this century, physicians accepted cholesterol levels as high as 250 as "normal." So it was a bit revolutionary in 1987 when the National Cholesterol Education Program, speaking on behalf of federal and private health groups, declared the following health goal: **All adults should maintain a total cholesterol level below 200.** A reading of less than 200 placed an adult in the "low-risk" or "desirable" blood cholesterol category. By age, the other NCEP guidelines are:

MODERATE RISK

Age	Cholesterol Level
20–29	200–220
30–39	200–240
40+	200–260

HIGH RISK

Age	Cholesterol Level
20–29	Over 220
30–39	Over 240
40+	Over 260

If everyone in the U.S. lowered his or her cholesterol reading to below 200, the death rate from heart attacks would plunge dramatically. So 200 makes a great goal for a national health campaign.

However, that doesn't make it the right goal for you. There is nothing magic or safe about a total cholesterol level of 200. A reading of 199 is by no means a vaccination against heart disease or a reason to ignore cholesterol.

Is There Any Magic Number?

There's no total cholesterol level that makes a person immune to a heart attack. However, Dr. William Cassells, head of the Framingham Heart Study, has said that he's never seen a heart attack suffered by a person with a reading of 150 or under. Although the average total cholesterol level of adult males in some areas of Japan is as low as 145, these levels are reachable only with a profound change in diet and lifestyle that relatively few Americans (myself included) are willing to undertake.

The risk begins to rise from extremely low level at about 160. People with readings from 181 to 200 have about a 30 percent greater risk of heart attack than do people with readings of 180 or less.

SEARCHING FOR A SILENT KILLER

One of the most frightening aspects of coronary artery disease is that it often produces absolutely no symptoms until a person suffers a serious heart attack or stroke. But now researchers are perfecting a new technique to detect closed arteries well before the onset of chest pain or more serious symptoms.

This procedure is called an arterial X ray, which is performed using a machine called an ultrafast CT. Doctors can detect the oldest parts of plaque clogging blood vessels, the plaque that has been deposited for so long that it has hardened. These deposits show up on the arterial X ray as tiny white spots.

Because it detects only hardened plaque, this procedure is most beneficial for patients age forty and older. From the amount of hardened plaque, doctors can estimate the amount of soft plaque that is further narrowing blood vessels. This soft plaque can often be removed when cholesterol levels are lowered through diet and lifestyle changes. For many patients, actually "seeing" buildup on the walls of their coronary arteries provides the incentive to overcome bad habits and adopt a more healthful way of living.

WHAT IF YOU'RE IN THE HIGH-RISK GROUP?

Research studies confirm that the NCEP is right on target with its high-risk category. The death rate from heart disease rises dramatically between 240 and 260. At 300, it's four to five times greater than at 200.

The good news for people in the high-risk group is that they receive the most benefit from small reductions in total blood cholesterol level. For example, a study done in Helsinki, Finland (one of the world's cholesterol capitals), tracked men with an average reading of 270. The results: An 8 percent reduction in blood cholesterol levels (to around 250) produced a 26 percent lower death rate.

TOTAL CHOLESTEROL GUIDELINES

The following guidelines on total cholesterol make good sense:

- Low Risk: Total cholesterol below 180
- Moderate Risk: Total cholesterol below 181–240
- High Risk: Total cholesterol over 240

4

LOOKING AT YOUR LIPOPROTEINS

•

Imagine that I had a suitcase full of $10 bills and $1 bills and counted out a stack of a hundred bills for you and a hundred bills for another person. You both would have the same number of bills, but you wouldn't know who was better off until you computed the number of $10 bills in your respective stacks.

In a similar way, just knowing your total cholesterol level doesn't enable you to calculate our total health risks. You also have to take a look at your lipoproteins to find out if you're better or worse off than someone else with the same total cholesterol level.

HDL—DEFENDER OF THE ARTERIES

I would be a sure bet to replace Microsoft's Bill Gates as America's richest man if I could find a way to bottle HDL and sell it as an elixir. Evidence is growing that HDL levels may be even a better predictor of the risk of coronary heart disease than total cholesterol levels. Making diet and lifestyle changes that contribute to an increase in the HDL cholesterol your liver produces is a vital step in adding years to your life.

Although we can't make HDL in a lab, we can measure it. Those measurements produce two meaningful numbers: the HDL level itself and the ratio of total cholesterol to HDL cholesterol.

The importance of the HDL level is highlighted by a study of about thirteen hundred patients who were treated for heart attacks at a Boston hospital. An amazing 40 percent of those heart attack victims had total cholesterol levels below 200—in other words, they were in the official low-risk category. But three-quarters also had HDL levels under 40, placing these people in the high-risk category. For those people, the HDL level was more important than their total cholesterol readings.

High HDL readings mean risk reduction. You're eight times more likely to have a heart attack if your HDL is 35 than if it's 65.

HDL CHOLESTEROL AND HEART DISEASE

The Framingham Heart Study found the following correlation between HDL levels and heart disease over a four-year period:

HDL Level	Men Developing Heart Disease (%)	Women Developing Heart Disease (%)
Below 25	18	
25–34	10	16
35–44	10	5
45–54	5	5
55–64	6	4
65–74	3	1
Above 75	0	1

YOUR TOTAL CHOLESTEROL/HDL RATIO

Your ratio of total cholesterol to HDL cholesterol goes hand in hand with your HDL level in assessing health risk. The easy formula for obtaining your ratio is:

$$\frac{\text{total cholesterol}}{\text{HDL}} = \text{ratio}$$

For example, if your total cholesterol is 200 and your HDL is 50, your ratio is:

$$\frac{200}{50} = 4.0$$

Studies have found a very strong correlation between ratios of 6.1 and above with coronary artery disease.

PUTTING IT ALL TOGETHER

The risk categories for HDL cholesterol levels and total cholesterol/HDL levels are easy to remember:

	HDL Level	**TC/HDL Ratio**
• Low Risk	Over 60	Below 4.0
• Moderate Risk	40–60	4.1–6.0
• High Risk	Below 40	Over 6.1

TOTALING TRIGLYCERIDES

As I discussed before, triglycerides are fats that the liver packages with cholesterol as VLDLs and sends off through the bloodstream to the cells. Common sense tells us that high levels of fat in the bloodstream are associated with a variety of health problems. But we don't know enough about the complex relationship between triglyceride and cholesterol levels to use the measurement of triglycerides as a definitive diagnostic tool.

So why do we bother to test for these little fat packages? Because we need use the triglyceride level to arrive at your LDL level.

We use the following formula to obtain the LDL level:

$$\text{total cholesterol} - \text{HDL} - \frac{\text{triglycerides}}{5} = \text{LDL}$$

This calculation is important because extra LDL cruising through your arteries is dangerous.

There's not a wide range between an acceptable level and too many. The risk categories for LDL cholesterol levels are:

- Low Risk: Below 130
- Moderate Risk: 130–159
- High Risk: Over 160

GENE THERAPY TO FIGHT DEADLY HIGH CHOLESTEROL

Less than 1 percent of Americans inherit hypercholesterolemia, a condition in which the body produces such huge volumes of cholesterol that LDL levels commonly reach 400 to 500 (130 is normal). Children born with this disease often die of heart attacks in their teens and early twenties. But now scientists are experimenting with brand-new gene therapy to counteract this condition.

In a procedure that seems more the stuff of science fiction than science, scientists remove about 15 percent of a patient's liver and nourish the billions of cells in lab dishes for about two days. Then the cells are exposed to a virus (the common cold virus has been used) that has been injected with copies of an LDL-lowering gene. The mixture of these liver cells and the virus is then injected back into the person's liver.

The preliminary results of a handful of these procedures have shown an average 20 percent drop in LDL cholesterol levels. Combined with drug therapy, patients have shown considerable improvement. Even more on the cutting edge are studies in which a virus containing a gene that raises HDL production have been successfully inserted into mice.

It will probably be decades before these techniques are perfected enough to become a staple of everyday medicine, but hope is on the horizon that cholesterol-related heart disease may eventually be conquered.

5

SUMMING UP YOUR CHOLESTEROL RISKS

In the last two chapters, I discussed four different risk factors:

- Total cholesterol level
- HDL cholesterol level
- Total cholesterol/HDL ratio
- LDL cholesterol level

With your cholesterol testing in hand, please circle your results in each of these four categories:

	Low Risk	**Moderate Risk**	**High Risk**
Total Cholesterol	Below 180	180–240	Over 240
HDL	Over 65	45–64	25–44
Cholesterol/HDL	Below 4.0	4.1–6.0	Over 6.1
LDL	Below 130	130–159	Over 160

Interpreting the results is easy:

If all of your results are in the low-risk column: Keep doing what you're doing. Unless you make significant—and harmful—diet or lifestyle changes, cholesterol is not a major health problem.

If one or more results are in the moderate-risk column, but none is in the high-risk column: You need to educate yourself about cholesterol and begin to make more sensible diet and lifestyle choices. The low-risk category is a reasonable and an attainable goal.

If one or more results are in the high-risk column: Reducing your cholesterol should be an immediate concern. After reading this book, you should consult with your physician about further testing and implementing a comprehensive plan to reduce your risks.

If you fall into the second or third category, don't panic—about three-quarters of all adult Americans are in the same boat. Instead, read on. In Part II, you'll learn why so many people have cholesterol problems and how to identify the cholesterol heroes and villains. In Part III, you'll learn how to make better diet and lifestyle choices that will lower your blood cholesterol levels, decrease your risk of coronary artery disease, and add productive years to your life.

YOUR CHANCES OF GETTING CORONARY ARTERY DISEASE

A study of eight thousand men age thirty-five to fifty-five over a nine-year period showed that the chances of having a heart attack were four times higher for those with total blood cholesterol levels over 268 than for those with levels under 194.

Blood Cholesterol	Heart Attack (%)
Below 194	4
194–218	6
219–240	9
241–268	11
Over 268	15

HOW FREQUENTLY SHOULD YOU HAVE FOLLOW-UP CHOLESTEROL TESTS?

If you are in the low-risk category, you can check your total cholesterol with a home testing kit every year and have a full lipid profile done every three years.

If you are in the moderate-risk category, you should check your total cholesterol every three months and have a full test every year.

If your are in the high-risk category, you should test your total cholesterol every three months and have a full test every six months until your risk level is reduced.

2

CHOLESTEROL—WHAT HURTS AND WHAT HELPS

•

6

WHY DO SO MANY OF US HAVE A CHOLESTEROL PROBLEM?

•

It doesn't seem fair that something our body makes, something that's essential to life, can also kill us. But since three-quarters of us have a cholesterol problem, we have to understand why so we can take the proper actions to correct it.

THE GENETIC LOTTERY

One of my dreams as a kid was playing in the N.B.A. But I didn't end up in that select 3 percent of all men who are 6'2" or over. So I ended up doctoring rather than dunking.

Most people are winners in the genetic lottery in at least one respect. You may be a math whiz, have perfect pitch, never need glasses, or be able to wiggle your ears. Or, you may have a digestive system that allows you to eat absolutely anything and never accumulate a speck of plaque on your artery walls. It doesn't seem fair that some people can efficiently get rid of any amount of cholesterol—but it's also not fair that Michael Jordan can hang in the air so long.

Unfortunately, the genetic lottery also produces some losers. A small percentage of people are born with few or no LDL receptors, a liver that overproduces cholesterol, or a liver that makes very few HDLs. These people can develop catastrophically high cholesterol levels and many die at an early age if there is no medical intervention.

The rest of us are in the middle. Most Americans—85 to 90 percent—are neither genetically immune to cholesterol problems nor genetically plagued by cholesterol levels that can't be controlled without medication. Where should you look for the reason for your less than ideal cholesterol levels? The bathroom mirror. *Your* diet and *your* lifestyle put you at risk for coronary artery disease.

CORONARY ARTERY DISEASE IS A CONDITION OF MODERN LIFE

Before you pronounce yourself guilty, let me act as your defense attorney. I'd argue that even though you did it (acted in a way that boosted your cholesterol levels), you shouldn't be convicted because you didn't know the difference between the right way to eat and live and the wrong way to eat and live. You were raised in an environment that practically guaranteed the eventual coating of some arteries. In other words, the real villain is modern life.

What do you think would happen if animals in the zoo were fed from the snack bar? Most of the hapless creatures would sicken and die if they regularly ate cheeseburgers, french fries, hot dogs, ice cream, and corn chips. We obey the "DO NOT FEED THE ANIMALS" signs because we understand that to survive in the unnatural habitat of a zoo, it's crucial that animals be fed a diet that takes into account their specific nutritional needs.

Our civilized world is in some ways an unnatural habitat for human beings. We are animals with a sophisticated body chemistry that has evolved over the seven and a half million years since our distant ancestors first ventured off on two legs. If the entire period of human evolution were a twenty-four-hour day, Big Macs, potato chips, cigarettes, fax machines, traffic jams, and escalators came into our lives less than a tenth of one second before midnight—a period of time that's far too short for our body chemistry to have adapted.

Then why do we live so much longer now? Drugs, vaccines, and medical technology have vanquished scores of humankind's traditional killers, greatly lengthening our average life spans. When it comes to fathoming the complexities of human body chemistry, we're at roughly the same primitive level that Galileo was when he first looked through his crude telescope at the stars. We basically understand how the major systems work, and we can treat specific systems. But so far we haven't come close to the comprehensive knowledge that would produce reliable cancer prevention or even a simple medical treatment for excess cholesterol.

THE FIRST STEP TOWARD A SOLUTION: UNDERSTAND EVOLUTION

The major tenet of evolution is: All living things physically adapt to their environment or they perish. By far the largest number of new species develop during times of great environmental change. One of those times was about 7.5 million years ago, when the climate of Earth cooled dramatically. The vast blanket of thick forests that had dominated the African landscape for aeons was replaced by broad, flat, grass-covered plains punctuated by stands of smaller trees.

One of the types of creatures most affected by this change were the apes who had found food and protection in the thick forests. Some species perished. But at least one ventured down out of the trees and moved out onto the plain, where it encountered one big problem—walking on hind legs and knuckles was too slow to escape from predators and too tiring to cover the distances required to gather food. The solution was a major physical adaptation—walking on two legs. Skeletal changes from a redesigned hip to shorter arms occurred, and over millions of years new species evolved.

By about 2.5 million years ago, one of those species had evolved to the point where it was identifiably human. *Homo habilis* had large brains, lived in groups, used tools, and perhaps even communicated with spoken language. Of most interest to us in learning about cholesterol, early humans had also developed a way of living that remained largely unchanged until the last few thousand years, what we call the hunter/gatherer lifestyle.

What this means is that these groups nourished themselves in two ways: hunting (or scavenging) for meat and fish, and foraging for fruits, nuts, berries, legumes, roots, and grains.

From a variety of evidence, from painstaking excavations of the debris around ancient campfires to careful studies of the few existing primitive hunter/gatherer societies, anthropologists have provided several relevant insights. Although meat was an important source of nutrients, foraging provided the bulk of our ancestors' diet. As much as 70 percent of their calories came from fruits, nuts, etc. Both hunting and gathering required a lot of exercise. The best guess is that hunters covered fifteen miles on foot on an average day. They roasted, boiled, or dried meat from game animals, which was much leaner than that of farm-raised animals we consume. For example, a venison steak has one-sixth the saturated fat of a comparable beef steak. Except in times of climatic upheaval such as prolonged droughts, their environments were bountiful enough to provide them with significant leisure time and were large enough to minimize conflict with other groups. The result was a life that was relatively stress-free.

ANOTHER GREAT ENVIRONMENTAL CHANGE—CIVILIZATION

After more than a hundred thousand generations, the last hundred generations have gone through the drastic transition from an isolated, self-sufficient rural society to an interconnected global urban one. The changes in our diet and physical activity level are profound. Food processing has taken fiber and nutrients and added sugars and fats. Food is eaten with sauces, condiments, coatings, and toppings. Our foods are often sautéed or deep-fried. Meat—much of it from fattened livestock—is inexpensive and readily available. Most of us expend a small fraction of the energy that our ancestors did to earn our food. From traffic to taxes, modern life tends to pile on stress.

There is no doubt that life today is vastly more comfortable than that of our ancestors. However, this environmental change has exacted a price that includes high rates of coronary artery disease.

DOES THIS MEAN WE SHOULD EXCHANGE OUR CONDOS FOR CAVES?

We couldn't go back to being hunter/gatherers even if we wanted to. The point of this brief anthropological lesson is to emphasize that high cholesterol is directly related to our diet and lifestyle. In order to lower our cholesterol—and thus lower our risk of coronary artery disease—we need to learn not only what things are bad for us but also what things are good for us. Then we can make more intelligent choices as we forage around the grocery store or hunt through restaurant menus. With intelligent choices, we can enjoy the benefits of modern life without paying too high a price.

7

THE CHOLESTEROL VILLAINS AND HEROES

Let's think of ourselves as heroes in an epic struggle to wrest ourselves from the clutches of coronary artery disease. Like any heroes, we first have to learn to recognize the villains—the major factors that contribute to higher total blood cholesterol levels, higher LDL levels, and/or lower HDL levels.

There can't be a happy ending if a story has only villains. Fortunately, in the quest for healthier arteries there are several heroes that can help along the way.

IDENTIFYING THE GOOD GUYS AND THE BAD GUYS ISN'T EASY

Research into the complexities of human body chemistry is extremely difficult. One important reason is that people can't be used as laboratory animals. We can't lock one hundred people in cages for a few years and give them diets identical except for one factor, such as the percentage of saturated fat, to see how that one variable contributed to cholesterol.

Instead we have to be like detectives building a case on circumstantial evidence. The collective medical establishment serves as the jury, weighing the guilt or innocence of any substance or habit. No one fact or study is conclusive. The accumulation of information over an extended period of time is the key.

I emphasize this point because it seems like every month a newspaper headline trumpets a study that supposedly names a revolutionary new cause or cure for cholesterol. My office staff handles dozens of phone calls from patients wondering if coffee really is the villain, or Vitamin E really is the answer.

Let's take coffee as an example for how fragmentary evidence can be misleading. A 1983 Norwegian study linked drinking of boiled coffee (but not coffee made with any machine that uses a filter) with higher cholesterol and triglyceride levels. Two other U.S. studies showed heavy coffee drinkers (five or more cups per day) had higher total cholesterol levels and a higher risk of heart attacks than people who drank no coffee. If you read these studies, you'd conclude coffee was a cholesterol villain.

But hold it a minute before you toss your Mr. Coffee in the trash. Other major studies—including the famous Framingham Heart Study—found no link between coffee drinking and heart disease. The studies that did show a link left unanswered extremely important questions, such as:

- Did the diets of coffee drinkers differ from the diets of non-coffee drinkers? For example, how much fat and cholesterol did they consume adding milk or cream to their coffee?
- Are heavy coffee drinkers more likely to smoke than non-coffee drinkers?
- Do heavy coffee drinkers lead more stressful lives than non-coffee drinkers?

Finally, the studies that implicated coffee exonerated other sources of caffeine, such as tea or cola drinks.

My conclusion is that the jury is still out when it comes to a link between coffee and cholesterol. I recommend that all my patients do everything in moderation, including drinking coffee. But I don't yet put it on my list of villains.

WHAT ARE THE CHOLESTEROL VILLAINS?

These are substances or conditions that have been proven to play a major role in the development of coronary artery disease by numerous research studies conducted over a long period of time.

Dealing with each villain pays immediate and significant dividends in reducing the risk of heart disease.

You have to watch out for five bad guys on your journey to good health:

- Dietary cholesterol
- Saturated fats
- Smoking
- Stress
- Obesity

WHAT ARE THE CHOLESTEROL HEROES?

Cholesterol heroes are substances or practices that have been shown to contribute to lowering overall blood cholesterol levels or improving HDL levels and HDL/total blood cholesterol ratios by numerous research studies conducted over a long period of time. Incorporating the heroes into your diet and lifestyle pay significant dividends in reducing the risk of coronary artery disease.

The good guys are:

- Polyunsaturated fats
- Monounsaturated fats
- Fish
- Exercise
- Soluble fiber
- Alcohol

IS A DIET OF RHEA IN OUR FUTURE?

Most of us can't imagine a diet without meat, a major source of cholesterol. After all, we humans have been carnivorous from the time our ancestors began to walk on two legs tens of millions of years ago. In the future, we may be able to indulge our appetites without ingesting the quantities of fat and cholesterol we do today, thanks to a group of pioneer ranchers.

On these ranches, the livestock is thundering around on two legs. That's because they're giant birds—ostriches, emus, and rheas. There are now more than three hundred such ranches across the U.S.

The meat of these birds is considerably lower in fat and cholesterol than even chicken and turkey. And there is a lot more meat per bird. Ostriches and their kin eat practically anything and are very inexpensive to raise.

However, a breeding pair goes for $50,000, and the meat sells for a hefty $20 per pound. But in the not so distant future, when herds proliferate, you might find yourself just as likely to sit down to roast emu as something that moos.

8

VILLAIN #1—DIETARY CHOLESTEROL

It doesn't take a doctorate in physiology to figure out that consuming too much cholesterol leads to higher blood cholesterol levels. However, everyone has a lot to learn about what the major sources of dietary cholesterol are.

WHERE DOES CHOLESTEROL COME FROM?

Remember, no plants produce cholesterol! You can consume all the vegetables, fruits, nuts, berries, grains, spices, vegetable oils, and other plant-related products you want and never, ever take in a gram of cholesterol—unless animal products were added in the food preparation (for example, butter on your baked potato). Conversely, every meat and other animal product contains cholesterol (unless that cholesterol has been removed during food processing).

WHICH HAVE THE MOST CHOLESTEROL?

Some foods have more cholesterol than others.

SOURCES OF CHOLESTEROL IN THE AVERAGE AMERICAN DIET	
Meat, poultry, fish	38%
Eggs	36%
Dairy products	15%
Animal fats	11%

Liver and Organ Meats

Since cholesterol is produced by the liver, it stands to reason that liver and liver products (such as pâté) are packed with cholesterol. So are other organ meats.

Brains

One reason cholesterol is vital to life is that it helps insulate our nervous system. The concentration of nerve cells in our brains means that animal brains have astounding amounts of cholesterol—almost thirty times as much per ounce as hamburger!

Eggs

All living things grow faster as embryos, which is why egg yolks are rich in cholesterol. This is also true of caviar, or fish eggs.

Milk and Dairy Products

Good mothers, human and animal, make sure their babies get plenty of cholesterol in the critical first two years of life. Whole milk, butter, and other dairy products made from whole milk have lots of cholesterol. As the fat is removed, the cholesterol content drops. For example, 2 percent milk has about two-thirds the cholesterol of whole milk, while skim has just a trace. Similarly, cheese, yogurt, ice milk, and other products made from lower-fat or skim milk have less cholesterol.

Fatty Meats

The rule of thumb for meats is easy—the more fat, the more cholesterol. Inexpensive cuts of beef have less cholesterol than those well-marbled T-bones. Chicken and turkey have less than beef, with skinless white meat much leaner than the dark meat. Other major offenders are spareribs, bacon, and luncheon meats like salami and headcheese.

HOW IS CHOLESTEROL MEASURED?

We measure cholesterol in food in milligrams, the same way we measure it in our bloodstream. The most useful way to look at the cholesterol content of food is to see how much is an average serving—for example, a 4-ounce hamburger, a pat of butter, a whole egg.

HOW MUCH DIETARY CHOLESTEROL IS TOO MUCH?

The American Heart Association and the National Cholesterol Education Program recommend consuming no more than 300 mg of dietary cholesterol each day. Since the average American's intake is 600 to 700 mg, cutting down to the guideline will help reduce total cholesterol and LDL cholesterol levels.

Again, however, 300 isn't a magic number. There's nothing unhealthful about cutting down to 100 mg per day.

9

VILLAIN #2—SATURATED FAT

I mentioned that much of the cholesterol in our body is packaged with dietary fats. So it's not surprising that our intake of fats affects all of our cholesterol levels. But the kinds of fats we eat have vastly different impacts on our body chemistry. One kind of fat is a major villain, while two other kinds wear white hats.

THE THREE KINDS OF FATS

Nearly all living things, plants or animals, contain some fat or oils. Fats and oils are compounds of carbon, oxygen, and hydrogen molecules that feel greasy or waxy, are tasteless and odorless, and are lighter than water.

There are three basic kinds of fats:

- Saturated fats contain the maximum number of hydrogen molecules they can absorb. Saturated fats are generally solid at room temperature.
- Polyunsaturated fats have fewer hydrogen molecules, but more than one. These fats are generally liquids at room temperature.
- Monounsaturated fats have only one hydrogen molecule. These fats are generally liquids at room temperature.

Almost every food we eat contains a mixture of these three kinds of fats.

WHAT'S SO BAD ABOUT SATURATED FATS?

Our liver uses saturated fats to make cholesterol, which means that we can't eliminate them completely from our diet. The problem is that most of us consume two or three times the amount of saturated fats we need. Like excess dietary cholesterol, excess saturated fat increases total cholesterol levels, LDL cholesterol levels, and triglyceride levels.

If you remember that saturated fats are solid at room temperature, it's easy to figure out that the fat in meat, egg yolks, cheese, butter, and lard is predominantly saturated. It's less obvious that milk contains saturated fat because it's homogenized—that is, the fat that floats to the top when milk is taken from the cow is broken up into such tiny parts that it doesn't separate.

THE TREACHEROUS TROPICAL OILS

The most dangerous saturated fat isn't connected with barnyards but with brilliant sunshine and sandy beaches. Coconut oil is the single most concentrated source of saturated fat, and palm oil is

SATURATED FATS

Substance	% Saturated	% Poly-unsaturated	% Mono-unsaturated
Coconut oil	87	2	11
Palm oil	82	4	14
Butter	66	4	30
Beef fat	52	6	42
Lard	41	12	47
Chicken fat	31	22	47

not far behind. What makes these fats so dangerous is that they're "hidden" in an astonishingly wide variety of prepared foods.

The reason these oils are used so much is that they are inexpensive and greatly enhance the flavor and texture of the finished products. If you read the list of ingredients, in cookies, crackers, cakes, powdered coffee creamers, and a wide variety of other prepared foods you'll find coconut and palm oils.

BEWARE THE WORDS "PARTIALLY HYDROGENATED"!

Many people use margarine instead of butter because it's made from vegetable oils (such as corn oil) that don't contain any cholesterol. The problem is that corn oil and other oils that are predominantly polyunsaturated fats are liquids at room temperature, and a puddle of margarine is very unappetizing. So food manufacturers solved the problem by adding hydrogen atoms to the polyunsaturated fats to make them behave more like butter. And because saturated fats are easier to use in cooking and add more taste, vegetable oils are also partially hydrogenated for frying or baking.

Partially hydrogenated fats also act like saturated fats by tending to increase cholesterol levels.

HOW MUCH SATURATED FAT SHOULD YOU CONSUME?

About 10 percent of your daily calories should come from saturated fats. Because dietary guidelines call for 30 percent of your total daily calories to come from fats, saturated fats should make up one-third of your fat consumption.

10

VILLAIN #3—SMOKING

Everyone knows that smoking causes lung disease. But you may not be aware that smoking is also a major contributor to the development of heart disease.

SMOKING LOWERS HDL LEVELS

The Framingham Heart Study showed that smokers had significantly lower levels of "good" HDL cholesterol than did nonsmokers. The lowest levels were observed in people smoking a pack or more a day of cigarettes, as well as in pipe and cigar smokers who inhaled. Remember, low HDL levels may be an even greater risk factor than high total cholesterol levels.

SMOKING ALTERS BODY CHEMISTRY

Smoke contains substances that are poisonous, so it's no surprise that smoking produces physical changes in blood vessels that make it easier for plaque deposits to form. At the same time, evidence is growing that smoking alters the chemical composition of the blood in a way that makes the formation of clots more likely. The combination of these two effects is a recipe for a heart attack or stroke.

SMOKING AND THE RISK OF HEART ATTACK

The Framingham Heart Study showed the following increases in the danger of heart attack to fifty-five-year-old men and women who smoked and had other risk factors:

- <u>Smoking cigarettes only:</u> Risk increased 56 percent for men and 71 percent for women.
- <u>Smoking cigarettes and high cholesterol:</u> Risk increased 116 percent for men and 165 percent for women.
- <u>Smoking cigarettes, high cholesterol, and high blood pressure:</u> Risk increased 221 percent for men and 336 percent for women.

IF YOU WANT TO STOP SMOKING...

You can obtain a Quit Kit, a packet of information that includes lists of local stop-smoking programs by writing or calling:

The National Cancer Institute
Cancer Information Clearinghouse
Office of Cancer Communications
Building 31, Room 10A18
9000 Rockville Pike
Bethesda, MD 20205
(800) 4-CANCER (except Alaska and Hawaii)
(800) 638-6070 (Alaska)
(800) 524-1234 (Hawaii)

GOOD NEWS—THE RISK EVAPORATES QUICKLY IF YOU STOP

If you stop smoking, your HDL levels will match those of a nonsmoker within one year—even if you've been smoking for decades. Although quitting won't scrape existing deposits from your arteries, it will begin to lessen your risk level almost immediately.

11

VILLAIN #4—STRESS

For most of us, having too much to do in too little time is a way of life. But scheduling every minute of every day can take years off your life.

Humans wouldn't have survived long as a species if we hadn't developed a strong physiological response to immediate danger. This "fight or flight" reflex gets our bodies ready for an intense burst of energy by flooding the bloodstream with hormones, such as adrenaline, which increase heart rate and respiration, elevate blood sugar, increase perspiration, dilate pupils, and slow digestion to make more blood available to the muscles. Stage two of this response is a mobilization of the body's repair systems to quicken clotting of wounds and removal of waste products from the blood. This reflex is responsible for many seemingly superhuman feats.

Unfortunately, it can also be responsible for several health risks. If the body remains on red alert for extended periods of time, we call this condition stress, and it's marked by constant tension, anxiety, or fear. For some people, stress is a short-term condition triggered by a single event ranging from a deadline at work to a death in the family. But for an increasing number of other people, stress is a chronic condition caused by the way they approach life, a lifestyle often called type A behavior. People who exhibit type A behavior tend to be overly competitive, aggressive, and harried.

STRESS AND BLOOD CHOLESTEROL LEVELS

Many studies have linked stress with an increase in total blood cholesterol levels. Elevated levels of cortisol, a hormone released into the bloodstream during periods of stress, are often found in people with high blood cholesterol levels. Adrenaline has also been tied to a faster buildup of plaque on artery walls. Other hormones may play a role in reducing HDL levels.

To make matters worse, ambitious, time-obsessed type A people are less likely to adopt lifestyle changes that decrease the risk of heart disease. They eat on the go, have fewer medical checkups, are more likely to smoke, and are less likely to get regular exercise. All of these bad habits are linked to higher blood cholesterol levels.

12

VILLAIN #5 — OBESITY

Almost half of Americans adults are overweight. This condition in itself is a risk factor for heart disease.

BODY FAT DETERMINES OBESITY

Surprisingly, what you weigh doesn't necessarily determine whether you're overweight. How can that be? Picture two 5'10" men standing side by side. One, a businessman who sits at a desk all day, weighs 200 pounds; the other, a football running back, weighs 220 pounds. Only the businessman is overweight.

The key factor in being fit or obese is the percentage of body fat we carry. Our bodies convert excess calories to fat. This fat is stored in certain parts of the body (parts with which most of us are far too familiar). The percentage of body fat can be calculated by using calipers to measure the thickness of certain skin folds.

Fashion models notwithstanding, zero body fat is not a healthy goal. Being underweight can cause changes in body chemistry (for example, women stop menstruating) that can cause health problems.

What's too much body fat? You should be concerned when your body fat reaches the 15 to 20 percent range. For most people, that occurs when their weight is about 30 percent above the desirable weight for their height, age, and build.

WHAT YOU SHOULD WEIGH

Below are the widely used tables compiled by the Metropolitan Life Insurance Company, based on data from 4.2 million life insurance policy holders. This table gives ideal weight ranges based on body type for men and women aged 25–59.

METROPOLITAN LIFE

MEN

Height	Small frame	Medium frame	Large frame
5'2"	128–138	131–141	138–150
5'3"	130–136	133–143	140–153
5'4"	132–138	135–145	142–156
5'5"	134–140	137–148	144–160
5'6"	136–142	139–151	146–164
5'7"	138–145	142–154	149–168
5'8"	140–148	145–157	152–172
5'9"	142–151	148–160	155–176
5'10"	144–154	151–163	158–180
5'11"	146–157	154–166	161–184
6'0"	149–160	157–170	164–188
6'1"	152–164	160–174	168–192
6'2"	155–168	164–178	172–197
6'3"	158–172	167–182	176–202
6'4"	162–176	171–187	181–207

WOMEN

Height	Small frame	Medium frame	Large frame
4'10"	102–111	109–121	118–130
4'11"	103–113	111–123	120–134
5'0"	104–115	113–126	122–137
5'1"	106–118	115–129	125–140
5'2"	108–121	118–132	128–143
5'3"	111–124	121–135	121–147

Height	Small frame	Medium frame	Large frame
5'4"	114–127	124–138	134–151
5'5"	117–130	127–141	137–155
5'6"	120–133	130–144	140–159
5'7"	123–136	133–147	143–163
5'8"	126–139	136–150	146–167
5'9"	129–142	139–153	149–170
5'10"	132–145	142–156	152–173
5'11"	135–148	145–159	155–176
6'0"	139–151	148–162	158–179

OBESITY AND BLOOD CHOLESTEROL LEVELS

One obvious reason that overweight people have higher blood cholesterol and triglyceride levels is that they eat more fatty foods. But evidence is growing that obesity is a separate risk factor by itself. Too much body fat appears to disrupt the process of producing and eliminating cholesterol, eventually accelerating the development of coronary artery disease.

SOME GOOD NEWS AND BAD NEWS

Studies show that even modest weight reduction can significantly lower blood cholesterol levels and the risk of heart attacks.

But beware of fad diets. Some low-carbohydrate weight-loss programs include foods with very high fat contents. You are likely to significantly increase blood cholesterol levels while losing weight. Equally dangerous are high-protein diets that often consist of packaged powders or liquids. Even fasting has been shown to increase blood cholesterol levels.

THE KEY TO LOSING WEIGHT

The only sensible way to reduce weight and *keep it off* is also the only sensible way to reduce blood cholesterol levels—learn how to make more intelligent lifestyle and dietary choices. In other words, learn what's good for you.

13

HERO #1—POLYUNSATURATED FATS

•

Chapter 9 explained that all fats aren't the same. Saturated fats definitely wear black hats in our saga. But their cousins, polyunsaturated fats, are essential to health and a positive factor in reducing blood cholesterol levels.

Polyunsaturated fats contain essential fatty acids—that is, fatty acids the body requires but can't manufacture. This is one reason that eliminating all fats from your diet isn't a good idea.

TWO IMPORTANT TYPES OF POLYUNSATURATED FATS

Scientists classify polyunsaturated fats by the location of the "missing" hydrogen atoms (remember, if a fat isn't missing any hydrogen atoms, it's saturated). The most common polyunsaturated fats are found in plant oils such as safflower oil, sunflower oil, corn oil, soybean oil, and cottonseed oil. The sixth carbon atom from the end in this type of fat molecule is missing a hydrogen atom, so it's called an Omega 6 fatty acid. I discuss this major source of polyunsaturated fats in our diets below.

The other important type of polyunsaturated fats is called Omega 3 (yes, the third carbon atom from the end is missing a hydrogen atom). Omega 3 fatty acids are primarily found in fish and shellfish. I discuss this type of polyunsaturated fats in Chapter 15.

POLYUNSATURATED FATS

Substance	% Saturated	% Poly-unsaturated	% Mono-unsaturated
Safflower oil	6	75	12
Sunflower oil	10	66	20
Corn oil	13	59	24
Soybean oil	14	59	23
Cottonseed oil	26	52	18

THE GOOD NEWS ABOUT OMEGA 6 POLYUNSATURATED FATS AND CHOLESTEROL

Numerous studies have shown that Omega 6 polyunsaturated fats decrease total blood cholesterol levels. According to Dr. Peter Kwiterovich, chief of the Lipid Research Unit of the Johns Hopkins University School of Medicine, every 1 percent increase in calories from Omega 6 polyunsaturated fat produces a decrease in blood cholesterol levels of about 1.5 mg/dl. The average American, who now gets about 5 percent of his or her calories from polyunsaturated fats, would see about a 7.5 mg/dl reduction by increasing that to 10 percent.

TOO MUCH OF A GOOD THING

As Omega 6 polyunsaturated fats lower your total blood cholesterol level, they also lower the levels of the beneficial HDL cholesterol. This means it's possible that your risk of heart disease would increase as your cholesterol level decreases.

You should replace saturated fats in your diet with polyunsaturated fats only until consumption reaches about 10 percent of your daily calories. That will give you all the essential fatty acids you need and produce a modest decrease in total blood cholesterol levels without any negative side effects.

14

HERO #2—MONOUNSATURATED FATS

If saturated fats are bad and polyunsaturated fats are good, monounsaturated fats are better. Although monounsaturates are the least common fats in the average American diet, they can play an important role in reducing coronary artery disease.

MEET THE MONOUNSATURATED FATS

One important insight into lowering cholesterol was gained from an investigation into the very low rates of coronary artery disease in Mediterranean countries. The Greeks, Italians, and Spaniards all cook with olive oil.

Olive oil contains predominantly monounsaturated fat. Numerous studies have shown that significant consumption of olive oil produces the same reduction in total cholesterol levels as polyunsaturated fats—*but without reducing HDL levels.*

In addition to olive oil the other significant sources of cholesterol-reducing monounsaturated fats are canola oil (a commercial form of rapeseed oil) and peanut oil. The use of canola oil has become increasingly widespread in recent years because, unlike olive oil, it lacks a strong flavor and doesn't burn during high-temperature cooking. If you've visited a movie theater concession stand recently, you've probably seen signs reading "Corn popped with canola oil"—a response to a widely publicized report of the high cholesterol content of corn popped in oils rich in saturated fats.

Using monounsaturated fats whenever practical is a wise step in reducing total cholesterol levels without reducing your good cholesterol levels.

MONOUNSATURATED FATS

Substance	% Saturated	% Poly-unsaturated	Mono-unsaturated
Olive oil	14	9	72
Canola oil	6	32	62
Peanut oil	17	32	46

15

HERO #3 — FISH

•

If you were looking for a group likely to have a high rate of heart disease, you'd almost surely pick Eskimos, who consume a high-fat, high-cholesterol diet made up almost exclusively of fish and marine mammals. But in fact, Eskimos have an unusually low rate of death from coronary artery disease. The reason is their consumption of fish.

FISH CONTAIN A MARVELOUS SUBSTANCE CALLED EPA

Many types of fish and shellfish are rich in a certain kind of polyunsaturated fat called eicosapentaenoic acid, or EPA. Because the third carbon atom from the end of these molecules is missing a hydrogen atom, it is classified at an Omega 3 fatty acid.

The initial source of EPA is the microscopic plant life called phytoplankton that is abundant in cold waters. The smallest fish eat the plankton, and they in turn are eaten by larger fish. EPA moves up the food chain until it's consumed by humans.

How Does EPA Reduce the Risk of Heart Disease?

Numerous research studies have shown that EPA has three very important effects in the body. First, EPA lowers total cholesterol, LDL cholesterol, and triglycerides by reducing the amount of

VLDL produced by the liver. At the same time, it does not reduce the amount of HDL cholesterol the liver produces.

EPA also inhibits blood clotting, reducing the risk of heart attacks and strokes in the same way that taking aspirin does.

Finally, EPA appears to chemically affect the LDL remnants in the blood, making them less "sticky" or less likely to adhere to the walls of arteries.

HOW MUCH FISH SHOULD YOU EAT?

The average American eats one-half ounce of fish a day (that probably means one tuna sandwich a week). One large study showed that increasing the average consumption to 1 ounce per day cuts the risk of heart attack by 50 percent. As a result, most experts recommend eating at least two 6-ounce portions of broiled or steamed EPA-rich fish or shellfish every week.

STAY AWAY FROM FISH OIL CAPSULES

Because we Americans love to pop pills, it is extremely important to emphasize that taking fish oil capsules is *not* a safe or effective substitute for eating fish and shellfish.

There is no evidence from any scientific study that fish oil capsules have the same positive effect as eating fish. Also, you'd have to take seven fish oil capsules to get the same amount of EPA in just 4 ounces of salmon. There is even some evidence that consuming a large number of fish oil capsules can cause negative side effects, such as flatulence and other digestive problems.

16

HERO #4 — EXERCISE

•

Daily rigorous physical exertion was an integral part of the lives of human beings for millions of years. The conveniences of modern life have made many of us sedentary creatures—to the detriment of our health. But the good news is that even a modest aerobic exercise program can produce significant health benefits.

WHAT IS AEROBIC EXERCISE?

Aerobic exercise is any activity that requires consuming oxygen over a period of time. Among the many activities that are aerobic are walking, jogging, swimming, dancing, cycling, skating, chopping wood, and mowing the lawn.

The opposite of aerobic exercise is anaerobic exercise, which is physical exertion done in intense bursts rather than over a long duration. Weight lifting and working out on Nautilus machines are anaerobic exercises that build muscle strength but do not reduce your risk of heart disease.

Who Should Exercise ?

Appropriate exercise programs are beneficial to nearly everyone, regardless of age or physical condition. Exercise is particularly beneficial to people who've had heart attacks or who have been diagnosed with heart disease.

Caution: If you're over thirty-five or if you are being treated for any medical condition, see your doctor before you begin an exercise program.

Benefits of Regular Aerobic Exercise

Within six to eight weeks of beginning to exercise regularly, your body benefits in several significant ways.

- Your body becomes more efficient at extracting oxygen from the blood, and your lungs can take in more air with every breath.
- Your heart can pump more blood with each beat, so it has to beat fewer times per minute.
- Your basal metabolism rate increases, which means you burn fat more quickly and efficiently.
- Your total and LDL cholesterol levels decrease, while your level of the good HDL cholesterol increases.
- Aerobic exercise improves what physicians call "collateral circulation." It improves the blood flow through arteries other than those narrowed by coronary artery disease, increasing total blood flow to heart muscles and reducing the risk of heart attacks even for people with coronary artery disease.
- Regular moderate aerobic exercise lowers blood pressure and reduces the tendency of the blood to clot.

How Much Exercise Is Enough?

You begin to reap benefits through moderate exercise (such as walking) for thirty minutes a day, four or five times per week. Chapter 20 describes exercise programs in detail.

> **WARNING—DON'T SMOKE!**
>
> Numerous studies have shown that smoking negates all the benefits nonsmokers derive from regular exercise.

17

HERO #5 — SOLUBLE FIBER

Every so often we open our newspapers to headlines that tout a new "miracle" cure for cancer, heart disease, or one of the other conditions that afflict a lot of people. Half a decade ago, the miracle of the month was oat bran, which was touted as the savior for those with high cholesterol.

Unfortunately, oat bran is not a miracle cure. But it is one of a number of sources of soluble fiber, a substance that can play an important role in reducing total blood cholesterol levels.

WHAT IS FIBER?

Fiber is material from vegetables, fruits, grains, and other plant food that human beings can't digest. There are two kinds of fiber.

- <u>Water-insoluble fiber</u> (fiber that doesn't dissolve in water) consists primarily of material from the cell walls of plants. Whole grains, wheat bran, and the skin of fruits and vegetables are rich sources of insoluble fiber.
- <u>Water-soluble fiber</u> is found in the flesh of fruits such as apples, oat and rice bran, legumes, and dried beans.

The average consumption of both types of fiber in the American diet has plummeted. The two main reasons for this decline are the removal of fiber in the processing of grains and other foods and the replacement of fiber-rich foods with high-fat foods such as meats and dairy products.

INSOLUBLE FIBER KEEPS THE DIGESTIVE SYSTEM HEALTHY

Insoluble fiber slows the movement of waste products through the intestines as it absorbs water from the intestine walls. People whose diets are high in insoluble fiber have much lower rates of cancer of the digestive system and other digestive diseases such as diverticulitis. High-fiber foods tend to be low in calories and high in nutrients, so they also are very useful in weight management. Among the best sources of fiber are breads, cereals and baked goods made with whole grains, wheat and oat bran, fresh vegetables (with skins), fresh fruits (with skins), potatoes (with skins), and beans.

SUPERFIBER IS ON THE WAY

Soluble fiber such as oat bran acts to lower blood cholesterol and fat levels because these grains have substances called "branch chains," formations of starches that wrap around cholesterol and triglycerides and carry them through the digestive tract without letting them enter the bloodstream. About one-fourth of the starch in oat bran is branch chains.

Now a group of Arizona farmers, supported by their state government, are developing a type of grain called Azhul barley that has twice the cholesterol-fighting power of any other grain. All of the starch in Azhul barley is branch chains, which means that all of it is available to wrap around cholesterol.

This wonder grain is under cultivation after years of laboratory work. If it proves hardy and economical to grow, it may become widely available on the market by the turn of the century. It can be used in breads, flours, and prepared foods, giving them an unseen but definitely appreciated anticholesterol power.

BENEFITS OF SOLUBLE FIBER

Like its insoluble cousin, soluble fiber is also beneficial to the digestive system. But it has one important additional benefit—it helps lower total blood cholesterol and LDL cholesterol levels. Researchers have found that soluble fiber increases the bile acids and LDL cholesterol that are eliminated from the body through the digestive system.

One reason soluble fiber isn't a miracle cure is that it is primarily effective only if it's part of a low-fat diet. You can't eat all the high-fat foods you want and expect fiber to flush the cholesterol our of your system.

Second, the benefits of a diet high in soluble fiber are relatively modest—an average 5 to 10 percent reduction in total blood cholesterol and LDL cholesterol levels. That makes soluble fiber a valuable part of an overall cholesterol reduction campaign but not a cure in itself.

MORE GOOD REASONS TO LOWER YOUR CHOLESTEROL LEVELS

Each year, 330,000 angioplasties are performed in the United States on people whose arteries are so clogged that they are in danger of having heart attacks. One procedure for opening clogged arteries is balloon angioplasty, in which a wire with a balloon at its tip is inserted into a leg artery, threaded up through the aorta to the coronary artery, and then inflated to compress the plaque on the artery walls. Any surgical procedure carries risks, but a new follow-up study of angioplasty patients provides yet another reason for making the commitment to lower your blood cholesterol levels through diet, lifestyle changes, and, if necessary, drug therapy.

Researchers have found that the angioplasty process may activate the cytomegalovirus, a virus that is present but normally inactive in about half of all adults. The cytomegalovirus can cause an excess of smooth muscle cells in blood vessel walls, which in turn leads to a very rapid reclogging of the arteries. Also, this hidden virus can mutate the gene that suppresses tumors, leading to an increased risk of cancer.

These adverse effects do not occur in all people. It's important to remember that angioplasties do save lives. However, it's also important to remember that most of us should take action now to decrease our risk of heart disease instead of waiting to be "rescued" by a surgical procedure.

18

HERO #6 — ALCOHOL

The white, waxy, fatlike substance that is the subject of this book was originally called "cholesterine." When it was subsequently discovered that this stuff was chemically similar to alcohol, the "ine" was changed to "ol" to make our modern word "cholesterol."

Perhaps the chemical similarity is the reason that *modest* consumption of alcohol contributes to coronary health. But like soluble fiber, alcohol is not a miracle cure. Indeed, it can be deadly in larger quantities.

A SENSIBLE APPROACH TO ALCOHOL

Regular consumption of a moderate amount of alcohol (2 ounces per day or less) has been shown to increase HDL cholesterol levels without increasing total cholesterol or LDL cholesterol levels. However, the increase is not as great as the increase in HDL levels associated with exercise.

Heavy consumption of alcohol is a major health problem in America. Too much alcohol can damage the liver, brain, nervous system, stomach, and pancreas. Heavy drinking can also increase triglyceride levels. Not to mention deaths from drunk driving.

Alcohol also can be dangerous even in small quantities when

RED WINE—A POTENT HEALTH DRINK

If you locked a dozen scientists in a well-equipped laboratory and demanded that they come up with a liquid concoction that would slash the risks of getting heart disease, cancer, and viral infections, they might be in that room for a lifetime and still not come up with a beverage as complex and effective as red wine. Recent research has found that red wine is a brew of at least one hundred antioxidants that protect against a wide variety of diseases.

One of the most powerful is a substance called calechin, which is also found in fruit, vegetables, and green tea. But no other food causes calechin in the bloodstream to soar to the levels seen in a person who has just drunk two glasses of red wine.

Why doesn't white wine have the same health benefits? The antioxidants are concentrated in the skin of the grapes, which are used in making red wine but not white wine. Calechin and other antioxidants also break down with age, so new red wines like Beaujolais are healthier than aged Bordeaux or Cabernets.

Before you fill the vegetable bin with bottles, remember that red wine, like all other alcoholic beverages, carries many health risks. People in the south of France, who drink lots of red wine, do have a low rate of death from heart disease, but they don't live significantly longer than Americans. Among their leading health problems are cirrhosis of the liver caused by heavy drinking, lung cancer, and other diseases caused by smoking.

If you enjoy red wine, drink it in moderation—a glass or two per day.

taken with a wide variety of over-the-counter and prescription medications, from cold remedies to ulcer medications.

Alcoholic beverages contain significant "empty" calories that may make it more difficult to lose weight. Even small amounts of alcohol can contribute to higher blood pressure.

Finally, alcoholism is a tremendous social problem that takes enormous financial, emotional, and physical tolls on those addicted to alcohol as well as their families.

I have a two-part recommendation on alcohol:

- If you don't drink now, don't start. The potential dangers if you find you can't handle moderate drinking far outweigh the modest health benefits.
- If you currently enjoy a glass of wine or beer with dinner and you don't have any alcohol-related problems, there's no reason to deny yourself this pleasure.

3

IT'S YOUR CHOICE—A
FLEXIBLE, SENSIBLE, TEN-STEP
CHOLESTEROL-REDUCTION PLAN

•

19

COMMIT TO A LIFETIME OF HEART-SMART CHOICES

•

You've assessed your risk of coronary artery disease and learned everything important you need to know about cholesterol and the factors that raise and lower it. Now it's time to implement a sensible, long-term plan to reduce your risk and add years to your life.

ARE QUICK CURES A FORM OF HEALTH CARE FRAUD?

By now, you understand that the risk of heart attack associated with cholesterol builds up over decades. No one is going to keel over after wolfing down a double cheeseburger with fries or a three-scoop banana boat with whipped cream. Nor does a serious problem develop if you totally let yourself go on a one-week cruise, a two-week European trip, or a four-week holiday season.

More important, no amount of food deprivation and physical exertion you inflict on yourself over a short period of time will significantly decrease the risk of heart disease that has built up over the years. All the books and articles that promise to "cure" a cholesterol problem in a few weeks or months aren't science. They are science fiction.

FAT CONSUMPTION, CHOLESTEROL, AND HEART ATTACKS

A study done for a conference on the health effects of cholesterol compared groups of Japanese men who lived in Japan, Hawaii, and San Francisco. The results graphically show the correlation among consumption of fats, cholesterol levels, and heart attack risk.

	Japan	Hawaii	San Francisco
Fat consumption*	16	34	40
Saturated fat consumption*	8	23	29
Average total cholesterol	181	220	237
Annual deaths per 1,000 from coronary heart disease	1.2	2.4	4.0

* as percent of total calories

YOU CAN BEGIN EXTENDING YOUR LIFE TODAY

Even though there is no quick cure for cholesterol-related problems, you can make a healthful choice today.

1. You can continue to make the same diet and lifestyle choices.
2. You can begin to make different, more informed diet and lifestyle choices that decrease the influence of the cholesterol villains and increase the influence of the cholesterol heroes.

Choice 1 has only one consequence if you are currently in a risk category: The buildup of plaque in your arteries will go on and your risk of having a heart attack will continue to increase.

Choice 2, on the other hand, produces one of three different results, all of which are positive.

- The buildup of plaque will slow even if you make only a small number of positive new choices. This slowing reduces your risks and may add years to your life.
- The progression can be stopped.
- The progression can be reversed, decreasing the plaque levels and increasing blood flow in your arteries.

CAN ATHEROSCLEROSIS REALLY BE REVERSED?

Yes. A number of reputable studies have shown that in a significant number of cases, long-term diet and lifestyle changes that result in significant lowering of total blood cholesterol and LDL cholesterol levels and raising of HDL levels do result in a reversal of plaque buildup in as many as a third of the patients studied.

CHOOSING A HEART-SMART DIET AND LIFESTYLE

We all know that accomplishing major goals doesn't happen overnight. For example, take building a retirement nest egg. First we establish a long-term goal. Then we decide on a budget in light of our current income and fixed expenses. Finally, we make daily spending choices that collectively determine how closely we stick to our budget.

Reducing the risk of heart disease is exactly the same type of process. We set a goal and "budget" the types of foods we can consume and the amount of time we can devote to physical activity. Then we make a number of choices every day that collectively determine how far we advance toward our goal.

Your goal is to bring your cholesterol levels into the low-risk category. As we discussed in Chapter 5, the goals are the following cholesterol levels:

- Total blood cholesterol: Below 180
- LDL cholesterol: Below 130
- HDL cholesterol: Over 60
- Total/HDL ratio: Below 4.0

These are *long-term goals*. What's important is not how fast you reach the goal, but that you make a little progress every day.

HEART-SMART BUDGETS

When we make up a household budgets, we concentrate on two major areas, one negative and one positive. On the negative side, we try to reduce our expenditures. On the positive side, we try to find ways to increase our incomes.

Reaching your cholesterol goals also requires concentrating on two major areas: reducing the negative effects of the cholesterol villains and increasing the positive effects of the cholesterol heroes.

Begin your cholesterol planning by dealing with the cholesterol villains:

- <u>Dietary cholesterol</u>. The American Heart Association recommends that you begin by reducing your consumption to 300 mg. per day. If you are not making satisfactory progress in six months, you should gradually lower that to 200 mg. per day.
- <u>Saturated fats</u>. Your total fat consumption should be no higher than 30 percent of your total calorie consumption, and saturated fats should be held to 10 percent or less. For the average person, that means 20 to 25 grams of saturated fat per day.
- <u>Smoking</u>. Stop smoking as soon as possible.
- <u>Stress</u>. Take steps to alleviate the causes of long-term stress in your life.
- <u>Obesity</u>. Reduce your percentage of body fat to below 15 percent and your weight to less than 20 percent more than the "ideal" weight for your height, frame, and age.

Next, move on to the cholesterol heroes:

- <u>Polyunsaturated fats</u>. Try to consume 10 percent of your daily calories in polyunsaturated fats.
- <u>Monounsaturated fats</u>. These "good" fats should make up at least 10 percent of your total calorie consumption and at least one-third of your total fat consumption.
- <u>Fish</u>. Eat at least two servings of fish high in EPA each week.
- <u>Exercise</u>. Do some type of aerobic exercise for thirty minutes a day, four or five days a week.

- <u>Soluble fiber</u>. Gradually increase your fiber consumption to 35 grams per day, concentrating on the major sources of soluble fiber.
- <u>Alcohol</u>. One or two drinks a day have a positive effect on HDL levels. However, if you don't drink, don't start. If you average more than two drinks a day, reduce your consumption.

The following chapters explain in detail how to make the daily choices that will allow you to stay within your "budget" and meet your long-term goal. Remember, no one can possibly make all the right choices every day of his or her life. But gradually, over time, making better choices will become a habit that will continue for the longer lifetime you'll enjoy.

20

YOUR EXERCISE OPTIONS

Becoming more physically active is the best single choice you can make—not only for your heart, but also for your total physical and emotional health. If regular exercise becomes a habit, you'll have a longer and more enjoyable life span.

ANOTHER LOOK AT THE BENEFITS OF EXERCISE

We already know that regular exercise raises HDL cholesterol levels, lowers total blood and LDL cholesterol levels, reduces blood pressure, and lowers the heart rate so the heart doesn't work as hard. Almost as important are the crucial roles exercise plays in taming two cholesterol villains—obesity and stress.

Everyone who needs to lose weight should know one fact: **Increasing physical activity is essential to losing weight and keeping it off.** Numerous studies have shown that a majority of obese people actually consume fewer calories than people close to their ideal weight. The reason that they are obese is that they are significantly less active than nonobese people. As a result, overweight people have a lower basal metabolism rate, that is, they burn fewer calories during any type of activity than do people who are not overweight. The prescription for losing weight and lowering body fat is regular exercise, which burns calories and increases the basal metabolism rate.

Exercise is almost a magic tonic for stress. Physical activity releases the tensions build up when the body stays on red alert for an extended period of time, leaving you mentally and physically refreshed.

WHO SHOULD EXERCISE?

Nearly everyone, from healthy twenty-five-year-olds to older people who have had heart attacks, benefits from an appropriate exercise program. **One caution:** Everyone age thirty-five or over as well as anyone with one or more coronary disease risk factors should consult with his or her physician before embarking on an exercise program.

Many people equate an exercise program with those hellish "two-a-day" football practices or the eighteen-hour-a-day grind of military basic training. But trying to do too much too soon is the primary reason people abandon physical activity. Remember, you're not preparing for a sports season or a war—you're making the decision to increase your physical activity for the rest of your life.

You don't have to change into a jogging suit and running shoes to begin the important lifestyle change. Among the ways to add physical activity:

- Park at the far end of the lot instead of right next to the door.
- Use the stairs rather than the elevator or escalator.
- Mow your lawn or shovel your driveway instead of using a service.
- Rake part of your lawn instead of using a blower.
- Wash your car instead of having it done at the car wash.
- Get off the bus or subway a stop early and walk the rest of the way.

The benefit of being more active isn't only the extra calories you burn but also the attitude you instill in yourself.

PLANNING A REGULAR AEROBIC EXERCISE PROGRAM

The real health benefits of exercise come from a regular aerobic program that you make an integral part of your daily routine. When you plan a program, you have to think about four factors:

- <u>Frequency</u>. How many times per week you'll exercise.
- <u>Intensity</u>. How hard you will exercise.
- <u>Duration</u>. How long you'll exercise each day.
- <u>Variety</u>. The types of activities you'll pursue.

Frequency

Studies show that the benefits of exercise begin to appear with a three-day-per-week program, but the most significant improvements result from exercise four or five times per week.

Intensity

The way to increase the strength of any muscle is to gradually increase the amount of work that muscle has to do. This holds true for the heart, your most important muscle. The measure of how hard your heart works is your heart rate, or how many times per minute it beats. You should begin an exercise program by gradually increasing the heart rate over your resting heart rate. The result will be a strengthening of your overall cardiovascular fitness and a lowering of your resting heart rate.

To calculate how intensely you should exercise, you first need to determine your maximum heart rate. Subtract your age from 220. For example, if you are 45 years old, your maximum heart rate would be: $220 - 45 = 175$ beats per minute.

At the beginning of your exercise program, you should pursue your chosen activity intensely enough to elevate your heart rate to 50 to 60 percent of your maximum heart rate. For example, if you are 45 years old, your heart rate should rise to: $175 \times .50 = 88$ beats per minute to $175 \times .60 = 105$ beats per minute.

Your goal is gradually to increase your heart rate during exercise to 75 to 80 percent of your maximum heart rate, which will sustain an excellent level of fitness.

You can measure your heart rate by holding a finger (not your thumb) on a vein in your wrist or neck, counting the beats for 15 seconds, and multiplying by 4. Another good check is that you are breathing noticeably harder than normal without being out of breath.

Duration

A good measure of how hard your body works during exercise is the amount of calories it burns. It's no surprise that you burn a lot more calories per minute if you're running or playing full-court basketball then if you're walking. But you probably will be surprised to learn that the health benefits of exercising less vigorously over a longer period of time are the same as exercising vigorously over a shorter period of time. In other words, walking or using a stationary cycle are just as beneficial to your heart as running or aerobic dance.

If you haven't been exercising regularly, start with a less vigorous exercise such as walking, slow swimming, or slow or stationary cycling. Start with ten minutes per day (at the starting heart rate you've calculated) three or four days per week. Gradually increase your duration in five-minute intervals to about twenty minutes per day after six to eight weeks and then thirty minutes per day by six months.

Over the long run, your goal should be to exercise sufficiently to burn at least 1,200 calories per week. The number of calories you burn during exercise depends on the physical demands of the activity and how much you weigh. For example, a 180-pound man who walks four miles per hour (one mile every fifteen minutes) burns 6.63 calories per minute. Let's figure out how long he needs to exercise to burn 1,200 calories: $1,200 \div 6.63 = 180$ minutes, or 3 hours. If he walks five days per week, he needs to exercise for thirty-six minutes each day.

Variety

Although you do have to exercise regularly, you don't have to pursue the same activity each time. For example, you could work out on a stationary cycle twice a week, walk twice a week, and play handball or racquetball on the fifth day. You can also vary your exercise program with the seasons, substituting bicycling in the summer for an aerobics class during the winter.

When changing activities, just keep two things in mind:

- Pursue the activity intensely enough to bring your heart rate to your target level.
- Adjust the duration according to the number of calories you are burning.

CALORIES BURNED DURING EXERCISE

Food is our bodies' fuel, and the harder we work, the more fuel we burn. Because it's harder to move a heavy object than a lighter one, the number of calories burned during any type of exercise increases with body weight. From the table below, you can get a good idea of how many calories you burn during various types of aerobic exercise.

		Weight		
Calories Burned During 20 Minutes of Exercise	**125 lbs.**	**150 lbs.**	**175 lbs.**	**200 lbs.**
Aerobics				
(moderate)	142	170	199	227
(hard)	227	272	315	364
Basketball	316	375	437	500
Cycling				
(10 mph)	156	188	219	250
(11 mph)	182	219	259	296
(12 mph)	213	256	299	341
(13 mph)	242	290	338	386
Dancing	170	205	239	272
Golf (pulling cart)	103	122	143	164

	Weight			
Calories Burned During 20 Minutes of Exercise	**125 lbs.**	**150 lbs.**	**175 lbs.**	**200 lbs.**
Handball	284	341	398	455
Ice Skating	165	197	230	263
Jogging				
(10-min. mile)	284	341	398	455
(12-min. mile)	242	290	338	386
(13-min. mile)	199	214	278	318
(14-min. mile)	170	205	239	272
(15-min. mile)	142	170	199	227
(17-min. mile)	113	137	159	182
Lawn Mowing	103	122	143	164
Roller Skating	145	174	203	207
Rowing	370	443	517	591
Running				
(5-min. mile)	512	614	716	818
(6-min. mile)	440	529	617	734
(7-min. mile)	383	460	537	614
(8-min. mile)	344	409	478	545
Skiing, cross-country	284	341	398	455
Skiing, downhill	229	272	318	364
Swimming				
(slow)	218	263	306	350
(fast)	267	320	374	428
Tennis				
(doubles)	142	170	199	227
(singles)	185	221	259	296
Walking				
(20-min. mile)	95	119	139	159
(26-min. mile)	85	102	119	136
Waterskiing	199	239	278	318

IMPORTANT REMINDERS FOR BEFORE AND AFTER EXERCISE

You can't just begin any exercise activity, no matter how mild, without stretching your muscles first. Without a warm-up, you face a serious risk of injury.

Also, don't sit down immediately after exercise. Blood pooling in the lower part of your body during any vigorous activity can cause nausea or dizziness if you don't stay on your feet for a five-minute cooling-off period.

SCHEDULE EXERCISE LIKE ANY OTHER IMPORTANT ACTIVITY

Exercise must become as routine a part of your day as showering and eating. If you don't think you have the time, consider this: 180 minutes of exercise is less than 2 percent of the time in a week. Make the choice to take this time for your health and your heart.

21

DECISION MAKING AT THE SUPERMARKET

•

Your success in lowering your cholesterol levels ultimately depends on what you choose to eat. However, it's a lot easier to make heart-smart choices if your refrigerator and shelves are stocked with heart-friendly foods. That's why the decisions you make in the supermarket are so important.

PLAN YOUR MENU BEFORE YOU SHOP

Researchers who study shopping habits have discovered that people who shop without a list tend to buy high-calorie and high-cholesterol foods. It's certainly not surprising that people who aren't heart smart are going to indulge in a lot more unhealthful impulse buying than people who know exactly what they are looking for.

This chapter takes you through the various departments of your supermarket and gives you some basic information about the foods you should be looking for. Chapters 22–25 provide further guidelines for planning three healthful meals per day plus snacks. Finally, you might want to purchase one or more of the cookbooks listed in Chapter 24 that contain a wide variety of heart-healthy menus.

When you're heart smart, you sit down to plan a week's worth of menus and make up a shopping list. It saves you a lot of time in the supermarket. And perhaps more important, having a refrig-

EAT LIKE A GREEK

A few years ago, with much fanfare, the U.S. Department of Agriculture unveiled its Food Pyramid, a graphic representation of new dietary guidelines designed to encourage Americans to adopt a diet lower in fat and higher in fiber. But a lot of experts don't believe that the USDA went far enough. In 1993, the Harvard School of Public Health, the World Health Organization, and a private foundation called the Oldings Preservation and Exchange Trust issued another food pyramid that they believe could more dramatically lower the incidence of heart disease all around the world.

These guidelines are called the Mediterranean Food Pyramid, which is based on the diet prevalent in Mediterranean countries. Harvard and the World Health Organization believe that the USDA Food Pyramid is too high in animal products and oils. The Mediterranean diet is much higher in plant-based foods. Plentiful are fruits, vegetables, and pasta, consumed with limited portions of yogurt, monounsaturated olive oil, and red wine.

Mediterranean countries have the lowest rates of death from heart disease of any of the Western developed countries.

---

erator and cupboards full of healthful foods makes healthful meal choices much easier.

THE NEW FOOD LABELS

Shopping for more healthful foods became a lot easier on May 8, 1994, when the Food and Drug Administration required labeling packaged foods with nutritional information that is easy-to-read and understand. Here's an example from a can of chicken rice soup with vegetables:

NUTRITION INFORMATION PER SERVING

SERVING SIZE	9.5 oz
SERVINGS PER CONTAINER	2
CALORIES	120
PROTEIN	8 g
CARBOHYDRATE	14 g
FAT	3 g
POLYUNSATURATED	less than 1 g
MONOUNSATURATED	2 g
SATURATED	1 g
CHOLESTEROL	20 mg
SODIUM	800 mg
POTASSIUM	160 mg

PERCENTAGE OF U.S. RECOMMENDED DAILY ALLOWANCES (U.S. RDA)

PROTEIN	15	RIBOFLAVIN	4
VITAMIN A	30	NIACIN	15
VITAMIN C	*	CALCIUM	2
THIAMINE	*	IRON	6

*Contains less than 2 percent of the U.S. RDA of these nutrients.

INGREDIENTS: CHICKEN BROTH, CARROTS, CHICKEN, POTATOES, CELERY, PARBOILED RICE, TOMATOES, DEHYDRATED ONIONS, SALT, FOOD STARCH—MODIFIED, SUGAR, HYDROLYZED VEGETABLE PROTEIN, MONOSODIUM GLUTAMATE, AUTOLYZED YEAST EXTRACT, GARLIC POWDER, SPICE.

Let's go through this label from top to bottom:

Serving size. This package provides nutritional information based on one serving of just over a cup. Evaluate the size of the serving carefully—it is sometimes unrealistically low to make the amount of calories and fat seem more acceptable. For example, most six-ounce cans of tuna suggest that they contain two and a half to three servings.

Calories per serving. One serving of soup has only 120 calories.

Fat and cholesterol. The soup contains 3 grams of fat per serving (note that fat is divided into polyunsaturated, monounsaturated, and saturated). The amount of cholesterol is 20 mg. per serving.

Sodium. Most prepared foods are high in sodium, and this soup is no exception. The 800 mg per serving is about all that is recommended for an adult *per day*. This is important if you are watching your blood pressure.

Vitamins and minerals. This soup provides about one-third of your daily vitamin A requirement, about one-sixth of your protein requirement, but not much else.

Is this soup a wise food choice? Accompanied by a tuna sandwich (not too much mayo!), you have a healthful lunch of about 450 calories.

UNDERSTANDING FOOD LABEL BUZZWORDS

These days it seems that every other product on the supermarket shelves has the word "light" or "lite" on the label. Most of us assume that "lite" means fewer calories or less fat—but that's not always the case. It can mean that the product weighs less, is lighter in color, or less dense. Occasionally, "lite" or "fat-free" products have more calories than their "nonlite" siblings. As a result, reading the nutritional label on the back is far more important than the label on the front.

However, several other words and phrases used on food labels do have specific meanings that can help you shop:

- <u>Extra-lean</u>. Must contain no more than 5 percent fat.
- <u>Leaner</u>. Must have at least 25 percent less fat.
- <u>Low calorie</u>. Each serving must contain no more than 40 calories or 4 calories per gram.
- <u>Low cholesterol</u>. Must have no more than 20 mg per serving.
- <u>Lower cholesterol</u>. Must have less cholesterol per serving than the regular product.
- <u>No cholesterol</u>. Must have less than 2 mg per serving.
- <u>Reduced calorie</u>. Must have one-third fewer calories per serving than the regular product.
- <u>Low sodium</u>. Must contain no more than 140 mg per serving.
- <u>Very low sodium</u>. Must contain no more than 35 mg per serving.

A Word About the List of Ingredients

Ingredients are listed with the largest quantity first. In this case, the soup's main ingredient is chicken broth. The only problem in the ingredients listed here is MSG, to which some people are allergic.

It's important that you take a look to see where the calories and fat are coming from. In particular, you should look for the following ingredients that may make a prepared food an unwise choice:

Bacon fat	Hydrogenated fat or oil
Beef fat	Lard
Butter	Meat fat
Chicken fat	Milk chocolate
Chocolate	Palm or palm kernel oil
Cocoa butter	Shortening
Coconut oil	Turkey fat
Cream	Vegetable fat
Egg and egg-yolk solids	Vegetable shortening
Hardened fat	Whole milk solids

RECOMMENDED DAILY INTAKE OF FAT BY CALORIE LEVEL

Calories per Day	Maximum Total Fat (g)	Maximum Saturated Fat (g)
1,000	33	11
1,200	40	13
1,400	47	15
1,600	53	17
1,800	60	20
2,000	67	22
2,200	73	24
2,400	80	26
2,600	87	28
2,800	93	30
3,000	100	32

SHOPPING IN THE PRODUCE DEPARTMENT

The fruit and vegetable aisles are the one area of the supermarket where you can fill your cart without worrying about fat or cholesterol. With the exception of avocados and coconuts (which contain fat), every choice you make will provide vitamins and soluble and insoluble fiber that will make you healthier and provide a greater feeling of satisfaction after a meal.

The following fruits and vegetables are the richest sources of soluble dietary fiber:

Apples (with skin)	Eggplant
Apricots	Figs
Beets	Onions
Broccoli	Pears
Brussels sprouts	Peas
Cabbage	Potatoes (with skin)
Carrots	Zucchini
Corn	

The produce department is also a good place to stock up onions, garlic, and herbs, which give food flavor without adding calories.

SHOPPING IN THE DAIRY DEPARTMENT

Dairy products provide 15 percent of the cholesterol in the average American diet, along with a hefty percentage of total and saturated fats. Smart shopping here is vital to a heart-smart diet.

Milk

Milk is an important source of calcium. Choose skim or 1 percent milk instead of whole or 2 percent milk.

Butter and Margarine

Just 1 tablespoon of butter has 33 mg of cholesterol and nearly one-third of your daily allotment of saturated fats. Margarine, which is made with vegetable oil, has no cholesterol—but it does vary widely in the type of fat it contains.

As mentioned, polyunsaturated fats and monounsaturated are liquids at room temperature. To give margarine a texture more like butter, the vegetable fats are partially hydrogenated, turning them into substances called transfatty acids. Stick margarine contains more partially hydrogenated fats than does soft margarine.

A few research studies have linked consumption of transfatty acids with higher cholesterol levels. However, the vast majority of experts still recommend using margarine instead of butter.

My recommendations are:

- Use soft margarine for toast, bagels, and other nonbaking needs.
- Use stick margarine for baking (soft margarine doesn't work well).
- Use a cholesterol-free nonstick cooking spray for frying.

Cheese

Almost all cheese made from whole milk is high in cholesterol and saturated fats. However, there are a growing number of low-fat or fat-free cheeses and cheese substitutes on the market. The American Heart Association recommends that you choose cheeses that have fewer than 3 grams of total fat and 2 grams of saturated fat per serving (usually 1 ounce).

Among the wiser choices are low-fat or nonfat cottage cheese, part-skim ricotta, and part-skim mozzarella.

Sour Cream and Cream Cheese

Regular sour cream and cream cheese are high in saturated fat and cholesterol. Substitute lite or low-fat sour cream and cream cheese.

Yogurt

Low-fat or nonfat yogurt is not only a good food choice eaten alone, but it also is a terrific substitute for sour cream. It can be served (mixed with fruit or spices) as a topping for baked potatoes, a dip for fresh vegetables, a spread on breads, as well as many other uses.

MEAT, POULTRY, AND SEAFOOD

This category accounts for nearly 40 percent of the cholesterol in the average diet. Your goal is not only to cut down on the quantity you eat but also to improve the quality of the meat, poultry, and seafood in your diet.

Meat

The "prime," or most expensive, cuts of meat are especially tender because they are heavily marbled with fat. Avoid the most expensive cuts of beef as well as:

- Organ meats such as liver, kidney, brains, and tongue
- Ground beef, rib roasts, and spareribs
- Pork spareribs, ground pork, and pork roast
- Sausage
- Smoked and luncheon meats
- Ground lamb and mutton
- Ground veal or veal breast riblets

Poultry

Chicken and turkey are leaner than red meat and should make up a larger portion of your diet. Turkey and chicken parts, especially white meat, are excellent choices. Ground turkey is a good substitute for ground beef. Avoid:

- Fatty fowl such as duck and goose
- Chicken livers, giblets, etc.

Seafood

Because many types of fish and shellfish are rich in EPA, nearly everyone can benefit from increasing the amount of seafood consumed. The fish highest in EPA are:

Anchovies	Perch
Bass	Rockfish
Bluefish	Salmon
Cod	Shark
Flounder	Snapper
Haddock	Swordfish
Halibut	Trout
Herring	Tuna
Mackerel	Whitefish

Most crustaceans and mollusks are low in fat and high in EPA. However, shrimp is so high in cholesterol that you should limit it in your diet. Crayfish and clams have relatively little EPA.

PASTA, RICE, POTATOES, AND BEANS

Most pasta—with the exception of egg noodles—contains little or no fat or cholesterol. Brown rice is a better source of fiber than white rice. Potatoes prepared with skins provide lots of fiber and vitamin C.

Beans and peas are among the very best sources of soluble dietary fiber, and they're also an excellent nonmeat source of protein. In order of fiber content, the products you should try to work into your diet are:

Black-eyed peas	White beans
Kidney beans	Butter beans
Pinto beans	Lentils
Garbanzo beans (chickpeas)	Lima beans
Split peas	

CONDIMENTS

Most condiments contain little or no fat or cholesterol. Using condiments instead of sauces and gravies can provide lots of flavor as well as significant health benefits. Caution: Choose lower-sodium versions of condiments such as soy sauce and barbecue sauce.

Among the condiments you should stock are:

Barbecue sauce	Mustard
Chili peppers	Picante sauce
Horseradish	Relishes
Hot sauce	Salsa
Ketchup	Soy sauce
Lemon juice	Steak sauce
Marinade	Teriyaki sauce

FATS, OILS, AND SALAD DRESSINGS

By definition, every choice in this category consists primarily of fats. Your shopping strategy is to purchase products that have little or no saturated fat. Your menu strategy is to use these products as sparingly as possible.

Fats and Oils

Avoid all products that are solid at room temperature, including lard and shortenings. Choose oils that are lowest in saturated fats and highest in monounsaturated fats, such as:

- Canola oil
- Olive oil
- Safflower oil
- Sunflower oil

Salad Dressings

The American Heart Association recommends choosing salad dressings that have less than 1 gram of saturated fat per serving. Many

French, Italian, Thousand Island, and blue cheese dressings exceed these recommendations. Fortunately, there are numerous low-fat or fat-free products available.

Another option is making your own salad dressing using olive oil or another recommended oil along with vinegar or lemon juice and spices.

Mayonnaise

One tablespoon of regular mayonnaise contains about 1.6 grams of saturated fats, slightly over the recommended level. If this size serving is enough for your tuna sandwich, it's acceptable. If your average serving is 2 tablespoons or more, choose a lite or nonfat mayonnaise.

PREPARED FOODS

The vast majority of boxed, canned, or frozen prepared foods are high in fat, sodium, and cholesterol. Read the labels extremely carefully. One important exception is tomato sauces that do not contain meat or other sources of fat.

CANNED FRUITS AND VEGETABLES

Fresh is vastly preferable, but canned fruits and vegetables can be more convenient. Just avoid:

- Vegetables packed in oil
- Vegetables with lots of extra sodium
- Fruits in heavy syrup

CANNED MEATS AND SEAFOOD

Avoid nearly all canned meats. Choose tuna, salmon, crab, and other seafood packed in water instead of oil.

DELI DEPARTMENT

A large majority of the meats, prepared salads, and other goodies offered at the deli counter are not good dietary choices. Stick with lean roast beef, lean turkey breast, and lean ham.

CRACKERS, BREADS, AND DESSERTS

You can avoid more saturated fat and cholesterol by reading labels in this category than you can in nearly every other section in the supermarket. For example, one brand of club crackers has 7 grams of total fat and 3 grams of saturated fat per serving. Another brand of club crackers has 2 grams of fat and .5 gram of saturated fat for the same-size serving.

The American Heart Association recommends crackers and cookies that contain fewer than 3 grams of fat and 1 gram of saturated fat per serving.

The American Heart Association recommendation for any kind of bread product, from bagels to tortillas, is fewer than 3 grams of fat and 1 gram of saturated fat per serving. Less-processed breads such as whole wheat, rye, pumpernickel, and oat bran contain more fiber than processed white breads.

Generally, avoid:

- Biscuits made with milk
- Cheese breads
- Cornbread
- Crescent rolls
- Croissants
- Egg breads and bagels

Fresh fruit makes a great dessert, but there are times when your sweet tooth demands something else. Unfortunately, you can load up on calories and cholesterol unless you're careful. Avoid:

- Prepared baked goods, such as pies, cakes, pastries, doughnuts
- Ice cream
- Brownies

- Cheesecake
- Puddings, custards, and mousses made from whole milk
- Snack cakes
- Shortbreads

Instead choose:

- Ice milk, sherbets, or low-fat or nonfat frozen yogurt
- Angel food cake
- Gelatin desserts or low-calorie puddings
- Cakes or muffins made from low-fat or no-fat mixes
- Low-fat or no-fat cookies

22

CHOLESTEROL-MELTING BREAKFASTS

•

I've found that making heart-smart choices for breakfast is easier and more immediately effective than making the right choices for any other meal. A good breakfast will jump-start your day and lay the foundation for a lifetime of better eating.

When one of my patients has a bacterial infection, I prescribe antibiotics to be taken every six or eight hours. Why don't I prescribe one big pill that could be taken once a day? Because antibiotics work best if there is a constant level in the bloodstream at all times.

Our bodies also work best if we provide a steady flow of nutrients over the course of a day. When we wake up in the morning, we've fasted for as long as twelve hours. A good, nutritious breakfast not only makes us more alert and energetic, but it is the best guarantee that hunger won't produce binge eating at lunch or dinner.

For most of us, mornings are hectic. Fortunately, there are more easy, quick, and healthful food choices for breakfast than there are for any other meal of the day.

THE HUMPTY DUMPTY DILEMMA

Americans on the average consume nearly three hundred eggs per year. Unfortunately, yolks are so high in cholesterol (275 mg each)

CHOLESTEROL AND FAT CONTENT OF BREADS, ROLLS, ETC.

Food	Calories	Cholesterol (mg)	Total Fat (gr)	Saturated Fat (gr)
Bread, white (1 slice)	63	0	1.2	.3
Bread, rye (1 slice)	70	0	1.0	.2
Bagel	190	0	1.0	.2
Biscuit	91	0	2.6	.6
English muffin	120	0	1.1	.3
Crescent roll	186	0	8.0	2.0
Hard roll	100	0	2.4	.3
Cornbread (4" × 2")	190	35	6.0	1.5
Cheese croissant	236	27	11.9	5.5
Pancakes, mix with egg (4)	230	72	5.9	1.6
Pancakes, light mix (4)	230	0	3.0	0

that eggs account for 36 percent of the cholesterol in the average diet.

The American Heart Association recommends limiting the consumption of whole eggs—including eggs used in preparation of baked goods and other foods—to two to three per week. You can, of course, use egg whites or egg substitutes to make omelets. But with so many other good breakfast choices, I think you should follow the AHA recommendations.

AVOID BREAKFAST MEATS

Bacon, Canadian bacon, and breakfast sausage are extremely high in cholesterol and saturated fats. Because you should limit your consumption of meat, poultry, and fish to 6 to 8 ounces per day, you probably want to save your allotment for lunch and dinner.

WATCH OUT FOR PREPARED AND FAST FOODS

Breakfast bars, toaster pastries, and instant breakfast drinks are convenient, but they also contain lots of fat and empty calories. It doesn't take much longer to pour cereal (be sure sugar isn't the first ingredient listed on the box) in a bowl or toast a bagel.

It's also tempting to pull up to the drive-in window of a fast-food restaurant—as long as you don't look at a nutritional analysis of your breakfast choices. An Egg McMuffin or a Burger King Croissant'wich contains lots of saturated fats and nearly 75 percent of your daily allotment of cholesterol. Don't trade nutrition for convenience.

DOS AND DON'TS OF A HEALTHFUL BREAKFAST

Breakfast is an excellent time to add fruit and fiber to your diet. Choose a menu that includes:

- 1 serving from the fruit group
- 1–2 servings from the bread, cereal, rice, and pasta group
- 1 serving from the dairy products group
- 1 serving from the fats and oils group

Fruit

All fruits are a good choice.

Choose:

- Melons, tangerines, strawberries, oranges, and apples are good sources of fiber.
- Apples, plums, peaches, pears, and bananas are good choices for eating on the go.
- Orange or grapefruit juice is a good source of vitamin C.

Cereals

Most cold and hot cereals are low in total and saturated fats and are cholesterol-free.

Avoid:

- Granola (many contain coconut or palm oils)
- Cereals with nuts
- Cereals with added sugar

Options:

- Bran cereals low in sugar and high in dietary fiber.
- Try sprinkling some oat bran on your cold or hot cereal.
- Sliced fruit sweetens cereal without adding empty calories.
- Instant hot cereals are easy to make in the microwave.
- Cinnamon makes hot cereals taste sweeter but has no calories.

Breads and Pastries

Avoid:

- All pastries, including doughnuts, sweet rolls, coffee cake, biscuits, and rolls
- Croissants
- Most commercially made muffins
- Pancakes and waffles

Choose:

- Whole wheat, rye, or pumpernickel bread (with soft margarine or jam, jelly, or preserves)
- Bagels
- Regular or whole wheat English muffins
- Homemade or low-fat bran muffins
- Pancakes made at home using two egg whites instead of one whole egg, skim milk, and polyunsaturated oil

Dairy Products

Avoid:

- Whole milk or 2 percent milk
- Cream or half-and-half
- Yogurt made from whole milk

- Cottage cheese made from whole milk
- Cream cheese
- Cheese (except low-cholesterol cheese)

Choose:

- Skim or 1 percent milk on your cereal
- Nonfat or low-fat yogurt
- Low-fat cottage cheese

Fats and Oils

Avoid:

- Butter
- Foods fried in oil, such as home fries

Choose:

- Soft margarine
- Nonstick cooking spray to grill pancakes

With Your Coffee

Some nondairy creamers contain coconut or palm oils that contain saturated fats. Read the labels and choose a product with no saturated fats. The best choice, if you don't like your coffee black, is skim milk.

CHOLESTEROL AND FAT CONTENT OF MILK AND DAIRY PRODUCTS

Food	Calories	Cholesterol (mg)	Total Fat (g)	Saturated Fat (g)
Whole milk (1 cup)	150	34	8.2	5.1
2% milk (1 cup)	121	18	4.7	2.9
1% milk (1 cup)	102	10	2.6	1.6

Food	Calories	Cholesterol (mg)	Total Fat (g)	Saturated Fat (g)
Skim milk (1 cup)	86	4	.4	.4
Butter (1 tbsp.)	108	33	12.3	7.5
Margarine, corn oil (1 tbsp.)	102	0	11.4	1.8
Margarine, safflower (1 tbsp.)	102	0	11.4	1.2
Yogurt, whole milk (1 cup)	139	29	7.4	4.8
Yogurt, low-fat (1 cup)	144	14	3.5	2.3
Yogurt, nonfat (1 cup)	127	4	.4	.3
Sour cream (2 tbsp.)	52	10	5.0	3.3
Sour cream, light (2 tbsp.)	35	8	2.0	1.2
Cheddar cheese (1 oz.)	115	30	9.5	6.1
American cheese (1 oz.)	106	27	8.9	5.6
American cheese, lite (1 oz.)	50	10	2.0	1.0
Mozzarella, part skim (1 oz.)	72	16	4.5	2.9
Ricotta, part skim (1 oz.)	39	9	2.2	1.4
Cottage cheese, creamed (1 cup)	218	32	9.4	6.0
Cottage cheese, low-fat (1 cup)	164	10	2.4	1.4

23

HEALTHY LUNCHES

A study of three hundred people who were trying to change their eating habits revealed that a majority found lunch the most difficult meal to plan. But even those of you who start dreaming about three-inch-thick pastrami sandwiches when the clock strikes noon can learn to make satisfying, and far more healthful, lunchtime choices.

AVOID LUNCHEON MEATS

One slice of beef bologna contains 90 calories, 78 percent of which come from fat. Half the fat is saturated. A sandwich with two slices contains nearly a third of your daily total fat allowance and nearly half of your saturated fat allowance.

Most luncheon meats—especially those that come in packages or cans—are also very high in fat and sodium.

WHAT ABOUT HOT DOGS, HAMBURGERS, AND PIZZA?

In 1992, according to the National Hot Dog and Sausage Council, the average American downed eighty hot dogs and two hundred hamburgers. Approximately 560 hot dogs were eaten each second, and McDonald's alone sold 190 hamburgers a second. These figures are so high that it seems almost un-American to recommend that

BAD BREATH IS BEAUTIFUL

All of us have been reading in recent years that garlic does a lot more than add zest to spaghetti sauce and ward off vampires. A recent study conducted by Dr. John Milner of Pennsylvania State University shows that a lot of the health claims made for this odoriferous food have a solid basis in fact.

Dr. Milner found that garlic (and related foods such as onions, scallions, shallots, leeks, and chives) are rich sources of sulfur-containing compounds that have a variety of pharmacological activities. Among the most effective are substances called saporins, which are steroidlike compounds. Saporins inhibit the formation of an enzyme in the muscle cells of arteries that contributes to the buildup of plaque and makes the arteries more prone to clotting. Garlic compounds also contain a variety of antioxidants.

The result, in one European study, was a lowering of cholesterol levels of 9 to 14 percent. Although the magnitude of those results has been questioned, evidence is growing that garlic and similar substances help lower cholesterol, lower triglycerides, reduce blood clotting, and even fight viral infections.

---

you exclude both from your regular diet. But they are loaded with fat and sodium—a single frankfurter contains 9 mg of saturated fat and 1,100 mg of sodium, and a large cheeseburger contributes three-quarters of your daily allotment of saturated fat and a third of your daily allotment of cholesterol.

Pizza is a better choice—if you lay off pepperoni, sausage, and other fat-laden toppings. Two slices of cheese pizza have twice the protein, 23 percent less fat, and 62 percent less cholesterol than a single McDonald's cheeseburger—and they are more filling. Pepperoni, however, nearly doubles the fat content. Low-calorie vegetable toppings—especially green peppers and broccoli—add nutrition without adding significant calories or fat.

HOW MANY CALORIES DO YOU NEED PER DAY?

To figure out how many calories you should be consuming per day, you need to use a figure that represents your "ideal" weight. If you don't know what you should weigh, take a look at the tables on page 54–5. Then classify your activity level (the amount of exercise you get) and multiply your ideal weight by the appropriate number to arrive at a daily calorie figure:

Sedentary   13 × _____ (ideal weight) = _____
Active   15 × _____ (ideal weight) = _____
Very active   17 × _____ (ideal weight) = _____

For example, if your ideal weight is 150 pounds and you lead an active lifestyle: 15 × 150 = 2,250 calories per day.

If your ideal weight is 150 and you are at that weight, a 2,250-calorie diet will maintain that weight. If your ideal weight is 150 but you weigh 175, on a 2,250-calorie diet you will lose about three pounds a month.

WHAT SHOULD YOU EAT FOR LUNCH?

You can choose from a wide variety of sandwiches, soups, and salads for a healthful lunch. Your ideal meal should include:

- 1 serving from the fruit group
- 1–2 servings from the vegetable group
- 1 serving from the meat, fish, and poultry group
- 1–2 servings from the bread, rice, and pasta group
- 1 serving from the fats and oils group

Sandwich Fillers

Sandwiches should be served on whole wheat, rye, or pumpernickel bread, hard or submarine sandwich rolls, bagels, or pita.

Avoid:

- Luncheon meats such as bologna, salami, pastrami, head-cheese, liverwurst, luncheon ham
- Canned meats such as Spam, corned beef, and deviled ham
- Deli salads prepared with mayonnaise, such as egg salad, chicken salad, ham salad, seafood salad
- Fast-food sandwiches such as hamburgers, cheeseburgers, fried fish, chicken cutlets
- Hot hero sandwiches such as meatball parmesan, veal parmesan
- Grilled cheese and other grilled sandwiches

Choose:

- Lean deli-sliced turkey breast, roast beef, or ham
- Water-packed tuna moistened with 1 tablespoon mayonnaise or diet mayonnaise
- Diced chicken or turkey breast moistened with 1 tablespoon mayonnaise or diet mayonnaise
- Low-fat cheese slices
- Sprouts, tomatoes, avocado, and other vegetables in pita bread

Salad Bars

Avoid:

- Shredded or diced cheese
- Diced ham or other meats
- Eggs
- Bacon bits
- Croutons, sunflower seeds, chow mein noodles
- Artichoke hearts or other vegetables marinated in oil
- Fruit in heavy syrup, such as peaches or pears
- Salads made with mayonnaise
- Salad dressings other than low-fat

Choose:

- Lettuce, spinach, cabbage, sprouts
- Vegetables such as broccoli, carrots, cauliflower, cucumbers, green peppers, mushrooms, olives, tomatoes, onions
- Garbanzo beans (chickpeas) and green peas
- Fresh fruit, such as watermelon, cantaloupe, and orange sections
- Low-fat dressings or oil and vinegar

Soups

The American Heart Association recommends that all servings of soup contain fewer than 3 g of fat, 2 g of saturated fat, and 20 mg of cholesterol.

Avoid:

- Creamed soups
- Soups with cheese
- Soups that don't meet the AHA recommendations

Choose:

- Most condensed soups made with water, including broths, bean soups, chicken soups, lentil soups, Manhattan clam chowder
- Minestrone and vegetable soups
- Some condensed soups made with skim milk or half skim milk and half water (check labels)

Fruit

Any fresh fruits or fresh fruit salads are good choices.

Pasta

Avoid:

- Egg noodles
- Pasta with cream or cheese sauces, such as fettuccine Alfredo
- Pasta stuffed with cheese or meat, such as manicotti, ravioli, tortellini
- Pasta with meat sauce, meatballs, or sausage
- Pasta salads with mayonnaise

Choose:

- Pasta with tomato sauce
- Pasta salad with diced vegetables moistened with olive oil or other acceptable oil and vinegar

Dairy Products

Avoid:

- Cheeses, except low-fat or no-fat cheeses
- Cottage cheese or yogurt made from whole milk

Choose:

- Low-fat cottage cheese
- No-fat or low-fat yogurt mixed with fresh fruit

24

NUTRITIOUS AND DELICIOUS DINNERS

Dinner presents both an opportunity and a danger for those of us who want to eat more sensibly. On the positive side, we normally have more time to plan and prepare dinner than we do the other meals of the day. On the other hand, studies have shown that a significant portion of people who overeat consume most of their calories in the evening. The solution: plan dinners that are healthful and satisfying.

CAUTION: DON'T GET TOO HUNGRY

One of the major causes of overeating at dinner is letting yourself get too hungry. Here are some solutions. Don't skip breakfast or lunch. No matter how busy you are, find time for a meal.

Drink plenty of water—at least eight 8-ounce glasses a day. You can substitute sparkling water or any other beverage that doesn't add calories to your diet.

Plan an afternoon snack. (Chapter 25 discusses sensible snacking.)

MAKE DINNER A SPECIAL OCCASION

We've learned that stress is one of the five cholesterol villains. Next to exercise, one of the best ways to counter stress is to set aside some time each day to relax and forget about the pressures and problems of daily life.

Many people find it very relaxing to make dinnertime special, even if they have only a half hour to set aside. Sit and relax before the food is served, even if it's for only ten minutes. You're less likely to eat fast (and thus eat more) if you don't rush into dinner.

Have a short "cocktail" party, even if you don't drink alcohol. Serve an appetizer of carrot and celery sticks, broccoli, green pepper, etc., dipped into nonfat yogurt seasoned with part of a package of dried onion soup or ranch dressing.

Sit down at the table instead of eating at a counter or in front of the television set. Use candles so dinner will be a "special occasion," even when you don't have company.

PREPARE FOOD SENSIBLY

We all know that a banana split or hot fudge sundae contains lots of fat and calories. That's why so many people are surprised when they eliminate these obvious diet busters from their daily menu and still can't lose weight or lower their cholesterol. One important factor is the hidden fat and calories we consume because of the way our food is prepared and presented.

For example, a cup of cooked broccoli contains lots of vitamins, no fat, and fewer than 50 calories. Just 1 tablespoon of butter melted on top triples the calories and adds one-third of our allotment of saturated fat. One 3-ounce fried chicken thigh contains three times the fat as 3 ounces of broiled sirloin steak. A 4-ounce serving of french fries has more calories and seventeen times the fat of a 10-ounce baked potato topped with ½ cup of nonfat yogurt.

The examples vividly show the dramatic impact of the "invisible" calories and fat. Pay as much attention to preparation as food selection when you're planning your dinner menus.

CHOOSING A MAIN COURSE

Our meat and potatoes diet is an American tradition. But those of us who want to adopt a heart-smart lifestyle should begin with a weekly schedule of main courses that includes:

CHOLESTEROL AND FAT CONTENT OF MEAT, POULTRY, AND FISH

Food (3 oz.)	Calories	Cholesterol (mg)	Total Fat (g)	Saturated Fat (g)
Lean beef	213	66	5.4	2.7
Prime beef	348	72	29.6	12.3
Ground beef	260	75	19.2	7.5
Beef liver	138	249	4.2	1.6
Chicken, white	142	72	6.6	1.9
Chicken, dark	174	79	8.3	2.3
Pork	271	77	20.7	7.5
Ham	156	45	9.0	3.0
Lamb	150	71	6.5	2.1
Veal	176	84	5.7	2.5
Turkey, white	114	55	2.4	.9
Turkey, dark	266	127	6.4	2.1
Tuna, canned (water-packed)	111	15	7.0	1.3
Flounder	99	58	1.3	.3
Trout	129	62	3.7	.7
Lobster	83	61	.5	.1
Shrimp	84	166	.9	.2

- 1 meatless
- 2 fish or seafood
- 4 meat or poultry

Meatless Main Courses

Among the excellent choices for meatless main courses are:

- Pasta (except egg noodles) with tomato sauce
- Pasta salad with diced vegetables and low-fat salad dressing
- Rice and beans
- Vegetable and rice casseroles

- Vegetable, split pea, or lentil soup
- Vegetable stew
- Eggplant parmesan made with low-fat mozzarella

Among the meatless dishes you should avoid are:

- Pasta filled with cheese or covered with cheese-based sauces
- Casseroles made with cream-based soups

Fish and Seafood

Chapter 21 listed the types of fish and seafood that are high in EPA and low in fat. However, the benefits of these foods can be negated by the wrong cooking techniques. The best ways to prepare fish and seafood are:

- Broiling (with lemon juice for moisture)
- Baking (with lemon juice for moisture)
- Poaching (in water, lemon juice, and/or white wine)
- Barbecuing (for tuna steaks, swordfish, shark, etc.)

Tuna, salmon, shrimp, crab, and lobster are excellent choices in casseroles made with pasta or rice. Fish and seafood stews and chowders (without cream) also make healthful and delicious main courses.

Poultry

The white meat of chicken and turkey contains less fat and less cholesterol than the dark meat. Also, the skin is loaded with extra fat. The best ways to prepare poultry are:

- Baking
- Broiling
- Poaching
- Barbecuing

Do not bread and fry or deep-fry poultry.

Poultry also makes an excellent ingredient for casseroles and hot or cold salads. However, if you have a hankering for ground meat, ground turkey is much more healthful than ground beef.

Meat

Chapter 21 provided tips on shopping for the leanest types of meat. Always trim all visible fat from meat before cooking. To tenderize the leaner cuts, marinate them for several hours in acidic liquids, such as tomato juice, vinegar, steak or soy sauce, wine, beer, lemon juice, or low-fat salad dressing.

The best ways to prepare meat are:

- Baking or roasting
- Broiling
- Boiling
- Barbecuing

Avoid frying or grilling meats.

You can extend the flavor of meat without adding extra fat and cholesterol by using small quantities in soups, casseroles, or stews.

BEANS, RICE, POTATOES, PASTA, AND BREADS

Carbohydrates are the foundation of our diet, providing energy, fiber, and a feeling of fullness that makes it easier to restrain ourselves from pigging out on fattier foods. However, as with meats, preparation is as important as selection of the carbohydrates you choose.

Beans

Beans are a great source of fiber—there are 13 grams in 1 cup of cooked lima beans. Serve beans with rice; add them to casseroles, soups, and stews; or put them on salads. Avoid pork and beans and prepared chili with beans, both of which are high in saturated fat and cholesterol.

Rice

Brown rice has about 30 percent more fiber than white rice. Avoid using butter or margarine on cooked rice or when preparing packaged rice mixes. Rather, use bouillon or tomato sauce to add moisture and flavor. Rice can also be used to thicken soups and stews.

Potatoes

Chapter 23 discussed baked potatoes as a lunch option; they are an equally fine dinner selection. Potatoes mashed with skim milk are acceptable, as are small potatoes boiled with their skins on. The latter can be sliced to make potato salad moistened with yogurt or olive oil or other acceptable oil.

Avoid french fried or home fried potatoes and packaged potato products such as au gratin or scalloped.

Pasta

As mentioned, pasta is a great main course choice. It's also an acceptable side course.

Breads

Rolls and breads, especially those made from whole grains, are excellent meal additions if eaten with little or no margarine.

VEGETABLES

The more vegetables, the better—if they're prepared properly. Whenever possible, steam vegetables (with the skin on) and serve seasoned with lemon juice, spices, or a little margarine. For salads, follow the recommendations in Chapter 23.

DESSERTS

The guide to supermarket shopping in Chapter 21 included a wide variety of desserts that fit into your heart-smart lifestyle. However, when planning your daily menus, you will probably find yourself choosing between dessert or snacks. In other words, if you want to indulge in a late evening snack, skip dessert. (For more information about snacking, see Chapter 25.)

HEART-SMART COOKBOOKS

Menu planning is easier with the aid of a cookbook that features low-fat, low-cholesterol recipes. Here are excellent volumes you'll find on bookstore or library shelves.

The American Heart Association Cookbook (Times Books, 1991).
The American Heart Association Low-Fat, Low-Cholesterol Cookbook (Times Books, 1989).
Choices for a Healthy Heart by J. C. Piscatella (Workman Publishing, 1987).
Cooking à la Heart by L. Hachfeld, B. Eykyn, and the Mankato Heart Health Program (Appletree Press, 1992).
The Fisher/Brown Low-Cholesterol Gourmet by L. Fischer and V. Brown (Acropolis Books, 1988).
Jane Brody's Good Food Book by Jane Brody (W. W. Norton, 1985).
The Living Heart Diet by M. E. DeBakey, A. M. Gotto, L. W. Scott, and J. P. Foreyt (Raven Press, 1984).
Low-Calorie Cooking by J. Shaper (Longmeadow Press, 1987).
Mediterranean Light by M. R. Shulman (Bantam Books, 1989).

25

SENSIBLE SNACKING

If you look at some diet books, you'll begin to believe that there was an eleventh commandment handed down that dictated "Thou shalt eat only three meals per day." For either physical or psychological reasons, many of us need to eat more frequently. If you make the right choices, snacking can easily fit into a heart-smart lifestyle.

SNACKING WITHOUT SNACK FOODS

The reason for snacking's bad name is readily apparent if you take a moment to glance at the selections available in the nearest vending machine. Chips, candy bars, nuts, and other offerings are among the worst food choices you can make. Only twelve potato chips contain a whopping 150 calories, 10 g of total fat, and 3 g of saturated fat. One 2-ounce candy bar has 280 calories and 14 g of fat. One ounce of mixed nuts has 180 calories and 16 g of fat. A package of cupcakes or cream-filled devil's-food cakes has 360 calories and 16–20 g of fat.

One of the best food choices you can make for your heart's sake is to give up traditional snack foods.

CHOLESTEROL AND FAT CONTENT OF COMMON SNACK FOODS

Food	Calories	Cholesterol (mg)	Total Fat (g)	Saturated Fat (g)
Potato chips (1 oz.)	150	0	10.0	3.0
Corn chips (1 oz.)	160	0	10.4	1.6
Tortilla chips (1 oz.)	143	0	7.4	1.2
Popcorn, butter flavor 3 cups)	100	0	6.0	1.0
Popcorn, air-popped 3 cups)	40	0	0	0
Cheese balls (1 oz.)	150	4	10.0	2.5
Club crackers (1 oz.)	140	0	6.0	2.0
Cheese crackers (1 oz.)	130	0	2.0	.5
Granola bar (1 bar)	130	0	5.0	4.3
Pretzels (1 oz.)	111	0	1.0	.5
Pork rinds (1 oz.)	150	24	9.3	3.7
Apple (1 med.)	80	0	.5	.1
Jell-O snack cup	80	0	0	0

HEALTHFUL SNACK CHOICES

Don't dismay, snackers! There are lots of tasty, nutritious options.

- Fresh fruit
- Dried fruit, such as raisins or figs
- Pretzels or air-popped popcorn
- Raw vegetables
- Low-fat or nonfat yogurt
- Low-fat or nonfat frozen yogurt
- Nonfat cookies or crackers
- Jell-O or low-fat pudding and custard
- Fruit juice
- Low-fat muffins

26

SAVVY MENU SELECTIONS WHEN DINING OUT

•

A survey by the National Restaurant Association revealed that the average American adult eats one out of every five meals away from home. Because restaurants offer more temptations than your cupboards and refrigerator, making intelligent choices when eating out can have a significant positive impact on your health.

DON'T BE A MARTYR!

It's important to emphasize one more time that the health risks from excess cholesterol build up over decades. You're not going to have a heart attack because you splurge on one meal or even on a seven-day cruise. The best way to ensure that you won't stick with your decision to adopt a heart-smart lifestyle is to treat making healthful choices as a kind of punishment that permanently deprives you of the pleasures of life.

Those pleasures include sumptuous meals at restaurants or in other people's homes on special occasions. If it's a birthday, anniversary, wedding, celebration of a promotion, or simply a reward for good behavior, go ahead and indulge yourself. The psychological benefits far outweigh any temporary (and probably minuscule) rise in your cholesterol level.

At the same time, don't treat every restaurant meal as a special occasion.

Anyone who's been on vacation has seen normally sedate and rational people act like idiots simply because they are away from home. Similarly, there are people who forget everything they've ever learned about nutrition the moment they're handed a menu. Although it's okay to splurge once in a while, you dine out most of the time because you're traveling, entertaining, or are too busy to get home to eat.

The problem, of course, as I mentioned above, is that most restaurant menus offer more temptations than your cupboards and refrigerator at home. Avoiding temptation begins with Rule #1:

Try to use the same criteria for making healthful choices in restaurants that you use at the supermarket or at home. For example, if you don't eat breaded and fried main courses at home, don't order them in a restaurant. Choose a baked potato over french fried or scalloped potatoes. Use oil and vinegar on your salad instead of bleu cheese or Russian dressing.

CHOOSE THE RIGHT RESTAURANTS

The menus in most fast-food restaurants are filled with high-fat and high-cholesterol offerings. Although acceptable menu options for the major fast-food chains are listed later in this chapter, you will find a greater variety of choices at restaurants that offer foods freshly prepared in a variety of ways. Through experience, you'll learn which restaurants offer the best selections. Whenever possible, choose those when you dine out.

STRATEGIES FOR DINING OUT

You'll find that even frequent restaurant meals will fit in perfectly with your choice of a healthier lifestyle if you follow these suggestions:

- Don't skip breakfast or lunch. You don't want to arrive famished.
- Begin with a small salad or a cup of soup, especially if others

in your party are ordering appetizers. If you get too hungry, you'll overeat.
- Try bread or rolls without butter. If they're tasteless, you're better off saving the calories than trying to make them palatable with margarine or butter.
- Limit yourself to one alcoholic beverage before the meal. Alcohol can stimulate your appetite.
- Order all salad dressings, sauces, and gravies served on the side and use them sparingly.
- Ask about low-fat options. Most restaurants are accustomed to such requests and they frequently have selections that aren't on the menu.
- Portions in restaurants are normally larger than those you serve at home. A good rule of thumb is to divide the main course in two when you get your meal and take half home in a doggie bag.
- Eat slowly and savor the food. The more slowly you eat, the smaller the quantity you'll consume.
- Order fresh fruit or sorbet instead of cake or pie. A second option is skip your before-dinner drink and have an after-dinner drink instead of dessert. If you absolutely can't resist, split a dessert with another member of your party.

HEALTHFUL CHOICES FOR ETHNIC DINING

Most of us find it a lot harder to evaluate types of food we don't prepare at home. Here are some suggestion for healthful choices in ethnic restaurants.

Chinese

- Hot-and-sour or wonton soup
- Steamed fish or dumplings
- Chicken, bean curd, or seafood stir-fried with vegetables
- Moo goo gai pan
- White or brown rice

Mexican

- Salsa
- Black bean soup
- Chicken tostadas
- Chicken or seafood fajitas
- Rice and beans

Italian

- Minestrone
- Linguine with red clam sauce
- Pasta with meatless marinara sauce
- Pasta primavera
- Chicken, fish, or veal in wine or red sauce

Japanese

- Miso soup
- Sushi and sashimi
- Chicken teriyaki
- Sukiyaki
- White rice
- Pickled vegetables

French

- Bouillabaisse
- Fish poached in wine
- Steamed shellfish
- Poached or broiled chicken
- Ratatouille

Greek and Middle Eastern

- Shish kebab
- Cucumber and yogurt salad
- Greek salad

- Stuffed grape leaves
- Couscous with chicken or vegetables
- Tabbouli
- Plaki

Indian

- Indian breads
- Raita
- Tandoori-style chicken and fish
- Biryani and pilaf

HEALTHFUL CHOICES FOR FAST-FOOD RESTAURANTS

Convenience, cost, and appeal to children are three reasons most of us end up eating at fast-food restaurants. It's very easy to consume more than a full day's allotment of cholesterol, calories, and saturated fats unless you're careful.

- Avoid all deep-fried foods
- Avoid beef and pork dishes
- Stay away from sandwich toppings such as cheese, bacon, and mayonnaise
- Don't order dessert

Following are menu suggestions for some major national fast-food chains:

McDonald's

- Hot cakes with syrup
- McLean Deluxe
- Chicken fajita
- Chunky chicken, garden, or side salad with vinaigrette dressing

Wendy's

- Plain baked potato
- Salad bar

- Small chili
- Caesar, garden, chicken, or side salad with fat-free French dressing

KFC

- Rotisserie chicken, white meat, without skin
- Corn on the cob
- Small mashed potatoes with gravy

Taco Bell

- Chicken burrito
- Chicken soft taco

Pizza Hut

- 1 slice Thin 'n Crispy medium pizza

Arby's

- Grilled chicken barbecue sandwich
- Light chicken or turkey sandwich
- Plain baked potato
- Chicken noodle soup

Burger King

- BK broiler chicken sandwich (no mayonnaise)
- Chunky chicken or side salad with reduced-calorie Italian dressing

Long John Silver's

- Baked chicken with light herb
- Baked fish with lemon crumb
- Shrimp scampi
- Light portion fish dinner
- Ocean catch or side salad

27

OPT FOR A STRESS-REDUCING LIFESTYLE

Of the five cholesterol villains, stress may be the most difficult to combat. The primary reason is that, as numerous research studies have found, we tend to deny or overlook the more undesirable facets of our behavior. We consider ourselves "competitive" rather than "compulsive," "conscientious" rather than "driven," and "self-assured" rather than "aggressive." Although we don't delude ourselves into believing we really didn't eat that three-scoop ice cream sundae, we commonly delude ourselves that we can handle any amount of stress.

SELF-DIAGNOSING STRESS

For most of the history of medicine, diagnosis was far more of an art than a science. Many symptoms such as fever or a rash can have hundreds of causes, and until the last three decades physicians often didn't know what really killed their patients until an autopsy was performed. Today, doctors have the benefit of sophisticated testing procedures and equipment that allow us to definitively diagnose hundreds of common diseases and conditions.

Unfortunately, science hasn't yet come up with a blood test for stress. But there are relatively commonsense criteria you can apply to yourself that can give you an idea if your stress level is high.

There are two common types of stress, each of which can be

diagnosed by different criteria: stress that results from life events that require significant lifestyle changes, and stress that results from a person's basic personality or overall pattern of behavior.

STRESSFUL LIFE EVENTS

Life events like the death of a spouse, divorce, or being fired from a job produce dramatic changes in our everyday lives. And numerous studies have conclusively linked dramatic change with high levels of stress. Two psychologists, T. H. Holmes and R. H. Rahe, developed a scale that rates life events in terms of the amount of readjustment and stress that they are likely to produce. The most stressful ten events on their Social Readjustment Rating Scale are:

1. Death of a spouse
2. Divorce
3. Marital separation
4. Jail term
5. Death of a close family member
6. Personal injury or illness
7. Marriage
8. Fired at work
9. Marital reconciliation
10. Retirement

Farther down on the list of forty-three events are such things as a change in residence, a change in jobs, a son or daughter leaving home, financial problems, or a change in hours at work.

There is growing evidence that stress caused by life events can lead to physical illness. Stress also places people at high risk of alcohol or drug abuse, depression, overeating, smoking, or other self-destructive behavior.

Coping with Stress Caused by Life Events

Studies have shown that the vital first step in coping with event-related stress is simply recognizing that a life event can have dramatic physical and emotional consequences. Unfortunately, denial is a common reaction even in the face of the death of a spouse or a child. The people who cope most successfully are those who expect life events to cause some stress.

People who realize that they are under stress can use the following strategies:

- Try to identify the feelings produced by the event and express those feelings.
- Understand that there is light at the end of the tunnel, that life will eventually return to normal.
- Take time arriving at decisions.
- Look at recovery as a long, ongoing process rather than believing that any one event (such as a funeral or the signing of final papers for a divorce) is a dramatic, official end to the event.
- Seek out support groups of people who are going through the same kind of life change.
- Seek counseling from a mental health professional.

PERSONALITY AND STRESS

A good deal has been written about the relationship between type A behavior and stress. A type A person tries to achieve more and more in less and less time. A type A may be competitive in situations that don't call for being competitive, impatient with slowness in others, talk fast and frequently interrupt, and quick-tempered and hostile. The demands a type A person places on himself or herself seem to produce a constant level of stress.

How can you tell if you're a type A? One clue is answering yes to many of the following questions:

Yes	No	I hate to wait in lines.
Yes	No	I become upset when my plans don't go smoothly.
Yes	No	I often find myself racing against the clock.
Yes	No	My work often infringes on my leisure hours.
Yes	No	My family, my boss, my spouse, and my friends expect too much from me.

Yes	No	It bothers me when my plans depend on others.
Yes	No	I do extra work to set an example for others.
Yes	No	When under pressure, I tend to lose my temper.
Yes	No	I try to do two things at once whenever possible.
Yes	No	I usually take work along on vacation.
Yes	No	When I make a mistake, it's usually because I rushed into something.
Yes	No	I often skip a meal to get my work done.

Type A Behavior and Heart Disease

Despite an enormous amount of research, there is still no conclusive evidence that type A people are especially disease-prone. However, certain aspects of type A behavior, such as hostility, irritability, and the need to dominate personal relationships, have been linked to increased risk of heart disease. Equally important, a significant percentage of the people who seek professional treatment for stress are the family members or close associates of type A people.

Few experts believe that a type A person can be changed into a type B person. However, the following techniques can help a type A person lower his or her own stress and the stress level of family members by modifying the most detrimental aspects of type A behavior:

- Avoid situations that evoke hostility, such as standing in long bank lines at lunchtime or driving at rush hours.
- Schedule work breaks such as going for a walk, browsing in a bookstore, or reading a novel.
- Take formal time-management training. Many companies have found that time-management training programs have given their employees a greater sense of control over their lives.
- Make a list of the types of behavior you'd like to change,

such as losing your temper or becoming too competitive in a social situation.
- Set up a regular exercise program. Exercise is a great stress-reliever—if you don't become compulsive about it.
- Learn relaxation techniques. Meditation, biofeedback, even prayer can significantly reduce stress levels.

28

DECIDE ON A LONG-TERM HEART HEALTH MONITORING PROGRAM

One last time, I want to emphasize that being heart smart is a lifelong process. Now that you've had your blood cholesterol levels tested, assessed your risk of coronary artery disease, and educated yourself about a heart-healthy diet and lifestyle, it's time for one more choice: **Decide to monitor your heart health for the rest of your life.**

YOUR PHYSICIAN IS YOUR PARTNER

One of the wisest steps to lifelong good health that anyone can take is to establish a relationship with a primary-care physician. A good primary-care physician (usually an internist or family practitioner) is your gateway to the health system and your partner in maintaining good health and preventing health problems whenever possible.

If you're one of the half of all Americans who don't have a primary-care physician, you should establish a relationship with one as soon as possible. The local medical society or hospital is a good source of referrals. Recommendations from friends and family members can also provide names for your list—but you should make the decision on your own.

It's difficult to compare the credentials of physicians if you're not an expert. However, you have every right to interview physicians to find one whose personality, hours, fees, insurance procedures, and office staff are most compatible with your needs.

CREATE A HEALTH MAINTENANCE SCHEDULE

It's important to see your physician regularly even if you're not sick. Your doctor will recommend a schedule for physicals and tests (blood work, X rays, EKGs, etc.) based on your age and physical condition. It's up to you to stick to the schedule.

The new home cholesterol tests make it easy for you to monitor your total blood cholesterol level. Once you've reduced your levels to the low-risk category, you should test yourself every six months or every year to monitor your overall levels. You should have a full lipid profile done every three to five years.

4

WHEN LIFESTYLE CHANGES AREN'T ENOUGH

29

CHOLESTEROL-LOWERING DRUGS

•

Lowering cholesterol through intelligent diet and lifestyle choices is the universally recommended first option for everyone in every risk category. But as a groundbreaking 1994 medical study proved, taking a cholesterol-lowering drug can be a lifesaving step for some people in high-risk categories.

TRY A DIET AND EXERCISE PROGRAM FIRST

Physicians usually advise that high-risk patients conscientiously follow a diet and exercise program to lower cholesterol readings for at least six months. Automatically prescribing medication is not appropriate in most cases. Cholesterol-reducing drugs normally have to be taken for a lifetime. When you stop taking a drug, your levels go back up. The most effective drugs are expensive. And any drug can have unpleasant side effects.

However, a significant number of patients at high risk can't succeed in lowering their cholesterol readings sufficiently despite their best efforts. There is new, dramatic evidence that these people should be taking a cholesterol-reducing drug.

CHOLESTEROL-REDUCING DRUGS

In 1994, the American Heart Association was presented with the results of a study of 4,444 men and women age thirty-five to seventy who had moderate to high cholesterol levels and who had been diagnosed with heart disease. Half the patients were given a cholesterol-reducing drug called simvastatin, while half were given a placebo. The results, in the words of Nobel Prize–winning physician Dr. Josepeh Goldstein, have "spectacular implications." The drug cut heart disease deaths in half, lowered "bad" LDL cholesterol by 40 percent and raised good HDL cholesterol. The drug also slashed the need for bypass surgery by 40 percent.

Dr. Michael Brown, another Nobel laureate, said, "This study will change medical practice." Dr. Suzanne Oparil, the president of the American Heart Association, said the study offered "definitive proof" that lowering blood cholesterol levels reduces the risk of heart attack and saves lives.

HOW DOES SIMVASTATIN WORK?

Simvastatin (Zocor) is one of four drugs on the market that are classified as HMG CoA reductase inhibitors. The other three are fluvastatin sodium (Lescol), lovastatin (Mevacor), and prevastatin sodium (Pravachol). They are called inhibitors because they block the production of an enzyme that the liver needs to produce cholesterol. When cholesterol production is reduced, more of the cholesterol already in the bloodstream is eliminated from the body, lowering total and LDL blood cholesterol levels. Patients taking these drugs, known as "statins," also experience moderately increased HDL levels. Statins are generally taken in tablet form once a day, with dinner.

HMG CoA reductase inhibitors have recently become the drugs of choice not only because of their effectiveness, but also because they have the fewest side effects for the vast majority of users. The most common minor side effects are headaches, rashes, indigestion, nausea, diarrhea or constipation, or muscle aches. In rare cases, they can affect liver function, irritate muscle cells, or interfere with kidney function. There are significant cost differences between the drugs in this category. You should discuss cost-effectiveness with your physician.

WHO SHOULD TAKE CHOLESTEROL-REDUCING DRUGS?

The new study focused entirely on patients who already had heart disease, not people who have high cholesterol levels but have not yet been diagnosed with heart disease. However, American Heart Association president Dr. Suzanne Oparil said, "As an individual, particularly if I were male and had a strongly positive family history [of heart disease] and a high cholesterol level, I would take it [simvastatin.]."

I believe that we physicians have to be more aggressive in prescribing cholesterol-reducing medications to patients who meet the following criteria:

- People who have heart disease; who have a strong family history of heart disease; or who have two or more risk factors such as obesity, high blood pressure, or diabetes, and whose total blood cholesterol level is 240 or higher and LDL cholesterol level is 160 or higher.
- People who don't have symptoms of coronary artery disease but have one of the above risk factors and whose total blood cholesterol level is 260 or higher and LDL cholesterol level is 180 or higher.

I want to emphasize, however, that anyone in any high-risk category should consult with a physician so that an individual evaluation can be made in light of individual health status and history.

OTHER COMMONLY PRESCRIBED CHOLESTEROL-REDUCING DRUGS

I have to emphasize that the simvastatin study does not mean that reducing cholesterol levels with other types of drugs won't have equally dramatic results. These other types of drugs, which tend to be significantly less expensive, are also options you and your physician may choose.

Bile Acid Sequestrants "capture" bile acids before they are reabsorbed by the liver so that they are eliminated from the body through the digestive system. Because the amount of cholesterol the liver receives is significantly lower, it makes more LDL receptors to capture more LDL cholesterol. The result is lower total cholesterol and LDL cholesterol levels. The two primary bile acid sequestrants are cholestryamine (Cholybar, Questran, and Questran Light) and colestipol (Colestid), both of which come as powders or granules that are mixed with some sort of liquid for consumption. They are both taken up to four times a day.

These medications have been used for more than two decades, and it has been shown that they have no major side effects. However, side effects such as constipation, abdominal discomfort, and a feeling of fullness are common. These drugs can also interfere with the absorption of other medications as well as folic acid and iron.

Nicotinic Acid, commonly known as niacin, is one of the necessary vitamins that we consume in our daily diet. However, when it is consumed in much larger than normal quantities, it acts on the liver to reduce the production of VLDL cholesterol and increase the level of HDL cholesterol. Niacin is available without a prescription, but *you should not take it in cholesterol-reducing quantities without consulting with your physician.*

In some cases, large quantities of niacin taken over a long time can interfere with liver function, cause gout, or affect vision. Common minor side effects include a feeling of warmth, flushing of the face, or general itchiness within minutes of consumption. Niacin can also cause stomach irritation and significant increases in blood levels of sugar in diabetics.

Fibric acid derivatives interfere with the production of triglycerides and VLDLs. Their main effect is to significantly reduce triglyceride levels, with an accompanying smaller reduction in total blood cholesterol levels.

The two major drugs in this category, gemfibrozil (Lopid) and clofibrate (Atromid-S) are taken in capsule form twice daily. They can affect liver function, increase the risk of gallstones, and, in rare cases, produce erratic heart rhythms and increased chance of blood clotting. Minor side effects include stomach irritation, diarrhea, muscle aches, increased appetite, and decreased libido.

Probucol (Lorelco) is stored in the fat cells of the body, where it actually enters LDL molecules and increases their elimination from the body. Because it's stored in the cells, it has to be taken for a while before it works and it lingers for as long as three months after consumption has stopped. Probucol decreases LDL and total blood cholesterol levels and can increase HDL cholesterol levels.

This drug, taken in tablet form twice a day, can produce irregular heartbeat. Common minor side effects include diarrhea, indigestion and flatulence, headaches, rash, and insomnia.

A FEW FINAL WORDS

I began this book with a fact and a promise. I'll end it with a guarantee: **Making heart-smart choices will have a profound positive effect on your emotional as well as physical health.** In other words, I guarantee that you will find following the suggestions in this book an emotionally uplifting experience. Keeping our house and car in tip-top condition gives us a sense of pride as well as preserves the value of these assets. But nothing is as important an asset as our good health. Time spent on living heart smart provides a sense of pride and self-worth that will give you renewed energy and confidence. Not only will you live longer, but you'll also increase your enjoyment of every single day.

APPENDIX 1

Cholesterol and Children

Unfortunately, children aren't immune from all the cholesterol problems that afflict adults. Evaluating their risk levels and instituting sensible diet and lifestyle changes while they're young can pay rich dividends in decades of longer, healthier life when they are older.

Army doctors who performed autopsies on the young soldiers who died in Vietnam found that nearly half of them had plaque buildup in their arteries. Other studies of children as young as age eight showed that about one in three children with a parent with high total blood cholesterol levels also had high total blood cholesterol levels. These studies also showed that children who had elevated cholesterol levels were extremely likely to have cholesterol problems and to develop coronary artery disease as adults.

WHICH CHILDREN SHOULD HAVE CHOLESTEROL TESTS?

Almost all doctors agree that children of a parent or parents who have total blood cholesterol, LDL cholesterol, or HDL cholesterol levels that fall into the borderline of high-risk categories should have their total blood cholesterol tested. Children whose parents or other close relatives have developed heart disease before age fifty-five should have a lipid analysis to determine their LDL and HDL levels as well as their total cholesterol/HDL ratios. This testing can be done as early as the preschool years.

Personally, I recommend that all my young patients have their total blood cholesterol tested by age eight to ten. The test is only a pinprick, and the benefits of being able to head off future problems far outweigh the minor discomfort and cost.

TEACH YOUR CHILDREN TO MAKE SENSIBLE DIET AND LIFESTYLE CHOICES

Even if you don't have your children's cholesterol levels tested, you should see that they make the same types of intelligent choices you do. It is particularly important to monitor the consumption of dietary cholesterol, saturated fat, and total fat while encouraging the inclusion of vegetables and fresh fruits. Habits of sensible eating and regular exercise formed at an early age tend to last a lifetime.

APPENDIX 2

CALORIE, CHOLESTEROL, AND FAT CONTENT OF SELECTED FOODS

	Serving	Calories	Cholesterol (mg)	Fat (g)	Saturated Fat (g)
Beef					
Chipped	3 oz	180	65	6	2
Chuck, pot roasted	3 oz.	243	81	17	4
Corned	3 oz.	213	83	16	5
Ground, regular	3 oz.	245	76	18	7
Liver	3 oz.	185	410	7	3
Roast, eye of round	3 oz.	225	64	7	3
Roast, rib	3 oz.	380	84	31	11
Roast, bottom	3 oz.	320	75	26	8
Steak, sirloin	3 oz.	360	74	25	8
Steak, T-bone	3 oz.	42r	80	38	14
Pork					
Bacon, Canadian	2 slices	86	27	4	1
Bacon	2 slices	93	16	8	2
Chop, loin	3 oz.	289	73	24	9
Ham, canned	3 oz.	160	66	14	5
Ham, cured	3 oz.	240	67	17	6
Tenderloin, roast	3 oz.	337	76	24	8
Spareribs	3 oz.	380	89	33	12
Poultry					
Chicken breast, skinless	3 oz.	140	73	3	1

	Serving	Calories	Cholesterol (mg)	Fat (g)	Saturated Fat (g)
Chicken breast, with skin	3 oz.	201	82	8	3
Chicken leg	3 oz.	156	78	6	2
Chicken liver	3 oz.	130	289	4	1
Duck, roast	3 oz.	140	88	12	5
Turkey, dark, with skin	3 oz.	201	85	8	3
Turkey, dark, skinless	3 oz.	186	79	7	2
Turkey, white, skinless	3 oz.	143	59	3	1
Turkey, ground	3 oz.	156	75	6	2
Lamb					
Chop, loin	3 oz.	240	80	12	5
Chop, shoulder	3 oz.	265	87	14	6
Leg, roast	3 oz.	160	72	8	3
Veal					
Cubed	3 oz.	172	128	4	1
Cutlet	3 oz.	187	127	6	2
Luncheon Meats/Sausage					
Bologna	1 slice	50	9	4	2
Bologna, beef	1 slice	90	20	8	4
Braunschweiger	2 oz.	205	88	18	7
Chicken roll	2 oz.	90	28	4	1
Frankfurter, beef	1	144	28	14	6
Ham, cooked	2 oz.	105	32	6	2
Salami	2 oz.	141	37	11	5
Sausage, pork	2 links	100	22	8	4
Sausage, pork patty	1	140	31	11	6
Turkey, bologna	2 oz.	122	44	10	4
Turkey, slices	2 oz.	75	42	4	1
Vienna sausage	2 oz.	190	32	16	8

	Serving	Calories	Cholesterol (mg)	Fat (g)	Saturated Fat (g)
Fish and Shellfish					
Catfish, breaded	3 oz.	200	69	11	4
Catfish, baked	3 oz.	125	58	5	1
Clams, raw	3 oz.	65	43	1	0
Cod, broiled/baked	3 oz.	90	50	1	0
Crabmeat, canned	3 oz.	60	59	1	0
Fish sticks	3 oz.	110	31	5	0
Flounder, baked	3 oz.	80	59	1	0
Haddock, baked	3 oz.	90	60	1	0
Lobster, boiled	3 oz.	100	100	1	0
Mackerel, broiled	3 oz.	190	60	12	3
Salmon, pink	3 oz.	119	34	5	2
Sardines, in oil	3 oz.	175	121	11	2
Scallops, broiled	3 oz.	150	60	1	0
Scallops, breaded	3 oz.	195	70	10	3
Shrimp, boiled	3 oz.	110	160	2	0
Shrimp, fried	3 oz.	199	141	9	3
Sole, baked	3 oz.	90	49	1	0
Trout, broiled	3 oz.	130	60	4	1
Tuna, in oil	3 oz.	240	36	18	3
Tuna, in water	3 oz.	105	36	1	1
Milk					
Buttermilk	1 cup	100	9	2	1
Evaporated	1 cup	340	75	19	11
Chocolate (2% fat)	1 cup	180	17	5	3
Cocoa (2% milk)	1 cup	236	20	6	4
Dried, nonfat	1 cup	245	12	0	0
Eggnog	1 cup	350	150	20	11
Milk (whole)	1 cup	150	33	8	5
Milk (2% fat)	1 cup	122	18	5	3
Milk (1% fat)	1 cup	110	15	2.5	1.5
Milk (skim)	1 cup	90	5	1	0
Cheese					
American	1 slice	90	25	7	4
American (light)	1 slice	70	13	4	3
Bleu	1 oz.	100	22	8	6

	Serving	Calories	Cholesterol (mg)	Fat (g)	Saturated Fat (g)
Cheddar	1 oz.	110	28	9	5
Cheddar (light)	1 oz.	80	20	5	3
Cheez Whiz	1 oz.	80	20	6	4
Cottage, creamed	1 cup	220	31	9	6
Cottage (low fat)	1 cup	90	5	1	0
Cottage, dry curd	1 cup	125	10	1	0
Cream cheese	1 oz.	100	30	10	6
Cream cheese (light)	1 oz.	60	10	5	3
Feta	1 oz.	75	25	6	4
Monterey Jack	1 oz.	110	30	9	5
Mozzarella (whole)	1 oz.	80	22	6	4
Mozzarella (part skim)	1 oz.	80	15	5	3
Muenster	1 oz.	105	26	9	5
Neufchâtel	1 oz.	80	25	7	4
Parmesan, grated	1 oz.	130	30	9	5
Ricotta (whole)	1 cup	430	125	30	20
Ricotta (part skim)	1 cup	340	75	18	12
Ricotta (nonfat)	1 cup	200	0	0	0
Swiss	1 oz.	105	15	5	3
Other Dairy Products and Substitutes					
Coffee Rich	1 oz.	40	0	2	0
Cool Whip	1 tbsp.	14	0	1	1
Cream, half & half	1 tbsp.	20	6	2	2
Cream, whipping	1 tbsp.	52	21	6	6
Egg, whole	1	80	213	6	2
Egg, white only	1	15	0	0	0
Sour cream	1 tbsp.	20	1	1	1
Sour cream, light	1 tbsp.	10	0	0	0
Yogurt, plain	1 cup	140	11	4	2
Yogurt, strawberry	6 oz.	216	11	4	2
Yogurt, low fat	1 cup	114	6	3	1
Fats and Oils					
Butter	1 tbsp.	100	31	11	7
Canola oil	1 tbsp.	120	0	13	1

	Serving	Calories	Cholesterol (mg)	Fat (g)	Saturated Fat (g)
Cooking spray	1 coating	6	0	1	0
Corn oil	1 tbsp.	120	0	14	2
Margarine, hard	1 tbsp.	100	0	11	2
Margarine, soft	1 tbsp.	100	0	11	2
Margarine, light	1 tbsp.	70	0	7	1
Margarine, sunflower	1 tbsp.	90	0	10	2
Olive oil	1 tbsp.	120	0	14	2
Peanut oil	1 tbsp.	125	0	14	2
Safflower oil	1 tbsp.	120	0	14	1
Soybean oil	1 tbsp.	120	0	13	2
Sunflower oil	1 tbsp.	120	0	14	1
Vegetable oil	1 tbsp.	120	0	14	1
Shortening	1 tbsp.	110	9	12	3
Salad Dressings					
Blue Cheese	1 tbsp.	60	5	6	1
French	1 tbsp.	60	0	5	1
Italian	1 tbsp.	71	0	7	1
Italian, light	1 tbsp.	6	0	1	0
Miracle Whip	1 tbsp.	70	5	7	1
Miracle Whip, light	1 tbsp.	45	0	4	1
Ranch	1 tbsp.	80	10	8	2
Ranch, light	1 tbsp.	20	0	1	0
Red wine	1 tbsp.	60	0	4	1
Thousand Island	1 tbsp.	60	5	5	1
Condiments					
Barbecue sauce	1 tbsp.	25	0	0	0
Cocktail sauce	1 tbsp.	15	0	0	0
Horseradish	1 tbsp.	10	0	0	0
Ketchup	1 tbsp.	15	0	0	0
Mayonnaise	1 tbsp.	100	7	11	2
Mayonnaise (light)	1 tbsp.	50	5	5	1
Mustard	1 tbsp.	14	0	1	0
Picante sauce	1 tbsp.	10	0	0	0
Relish, sweet	1 tbsp.	20	0	0	0

	Serving	Calories	Cholesterol (mg)	Fat (g)	Saturated Fat (g)
Salsa	1 tbsp.	5	0	0	0
Soy sauce	1 tbsp.	11	0	0	0
Sweet & sour sauce	1 tbsp.	26	0	0	0
Tabasco sauce	1 tsp.	0	0	0	0
Tartar sauce	1 tbsp.	72	5	8	1
Vinegar, wine	1 tbsp.	2	0	0	0

Breads and Rolls

	Serving	Calories	Cholesterol (mg)	Fat (g)	Saturated Fat (g)
Bagel	1	180	0	2	1
Biscuits	1	100	1	5	1
Breadsticks	1	100	0	2	1
Bread crumbs	1 cup	376	6	6	2
Cracked wheat	1 slice	65	0	2	1
Croissant	1	235	14	12	5
Dinner rolls	1	85	0	2	1
English muffin	1	130	0	1	0
French	1 slice	100	0	1	0
Hamburger bun	1	115	0	2	0
Hard roll	1	155	0	2	0
Hero/sub roll	1	390	0	8	2
Hot dog bun	1	115	0	2	0
Italian	1 slice	87	0	0	0
Muffin, blueberry	1	144	44	6	1
Muffin, bran	1	170	30	6	1
Oat bran	1 slice	70	0	0	0
Pancakes	3 average	190	55	7	2
Pita	1	155	0	1	0
Pumpernickel	1 slice	80	0	1	0
Rye	1 slice	70	0	1	0
Stuffing	1 cup	400	65	25	5
Taco shell	1	70	0	3	0
Tortilla, corn	1	55	0	0	0
Tortilla, flour	1	80	0	2	0
Waffles	1	90	1	3	1
Whole wheat	1 slice	70	0	1	0
White	1 slice	70	0	1	0

	Serving	Calories	Cholesterol (mg)	Fat (g)	Saturated Fat (g)
Candy and Chocolate					
Almond Joy	1 bar	250	0	14	7
Baby Ruth	1 bar	290	0	14	8
Butterfinger	1 bar	280	0	12	5
Caramels	4	120	0	4	0
Chocolate chips	½ cup	400	0	24	14
Chocolate sauce	1 tbsp.	50	0	8	2
Chocolate, semisweet	1 oz.	140	0	15	8
Chocolate, unsweetened	1 oz.	140	0	15	8
Fudge	1 oz.	115	1	3	1
Hard candy	1 oz.	110	0	0	0
Jelly beans	1 oz.	110	0	0	0
Kisses, chocolate	4	105	4	8	3
Kit Kat	1 oz.	165	7	8	5
M&Ms, plain	1 oz.	140	2	6	2
M&Ms, peanut	1 oz.	150	2	7	3
Milk chocolate	1 oz.	150	5	9	5
Marshmallows	4	100	0	0	0
Peanut brittle	1 oz.	130	0	5	1
Snickers	1 bar	280	3	12	8
Beans and Peas					
Bean curd (tofu)	2 oz.	82	0	5	0
Black	1 cup	225	0	1	0
Black-eyed peas	1 cup	190	0	1	0
Garbanzo beans (chickpeas)	1 cup	270	0	4	0
Lentils	1 cup	215	0	1	0
Lima	1 cup	188	0	1	0
Pinto	1 cup	234	0	1	0
Pork and beans	1 cup	225	0	1	0
Red kidney	1 cup	215	0	1	0
Refried	1 cup	285	16	2	0
Split peas	1 cup	230	0	1	0
Sprouts	1 cup	30	0	0	0

	Serving	Calories	Cholesterol (mg)	Fat (g)	Saturated Fat (g)
Nuts and Seeds					
Almonds, whole	1 oz.	165	0	15	1
Cashews, dry roasted	1 oz.	160	0	0	0
Cashews, oil roasted	1 oz.	160	0	13	1
Coconut, shredded	1 oz.	157	0	11	8
Macadamias	1 oz.	197	0	21	3
Peanut butter	2 tbsp.	190	0	17	3
Peanuts, dry roasted	1 oz.	160	0	14	2
Peanuts, oil roasted	1 oz.	160	0	20	4
Pecans	1 oz.	196	0	20	3
Sesame	1 tbsp.	45	0	4	1
Sunflower	1 oz.	160	0	14	2
Pistachios	1 oz.	170	0	15	2
Walnuts, black	1 oz.	179	0	16	3
Pasta and Rice					
Egg noodles, dry	2 oz.	210	55	3	1
Linguine, dry	3 oz.	250	0	3	0
Macaroni	1 cup	155	0	1	0
Noodles, chow mein	1 cup	220	5	11	2
Rice, brown, cooked	1 cup	230	0	1	0
Rice, white, cooked	1 cup	185	0	0	0
Spaghetti, cooked	1 cup	155	0	1	0

Fruits and Vegetables

Fruits and vegetables contain no cholesterol and no fats, with two exceptions—coconut and avocados.